TARA COSTELLO

RED MOON GANG

AN INCLUSIVE GUIDE TO PERIODS

ILLUSTRATED BY MARY PURDIE

PRESTEL
MUNICH · LONDON · NEW YORK

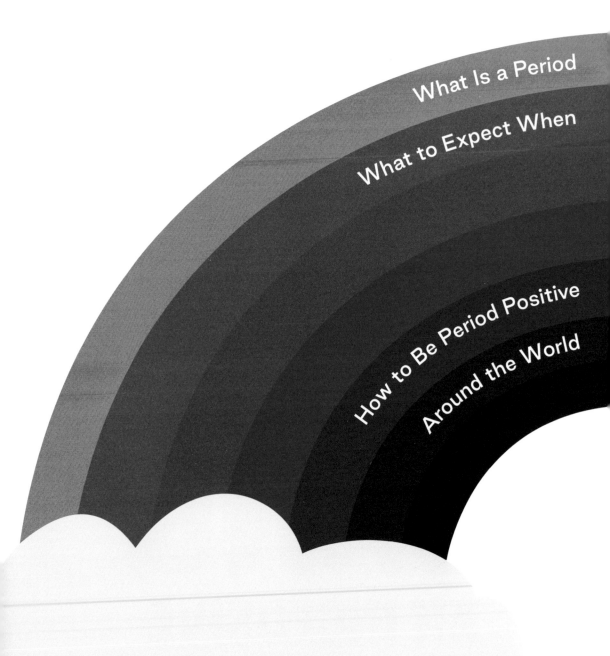

Introduction

Growing up, I absolutely hated having a period. I saw it as an inconvenience. Nobody told me it was something that could be managed, or an experience I could make better for myself. My first one happened when I was 11; my mum somehow knew it was coming. Although it was expected, it was still a shock to the system. It was hard to navigate, very bloody and also extremely painful.

From then on I was taught to be prepared for my period to turn up without a moment's notice and always carry pads (Fig. 1) with me. Looking back, this instilled in me a sense of fear. That said, my mum was pretty good at normalizing those sorts of discussions; when your seven-year-old won't stop asking you what a penis is, it not only forces you to have 'The Talk' several years earlier than you expected, but means nothing is off limits! While that was great, and I always felt like I could turn to her with any questions, a lot of negative influences were still present. There was so much out there that made me feel like I had to keep my period secret. Some of my most vivid and earliest memories of menstruation involve delaying plans, worrying about bloodstains and skipping school. Little did I know that these experiences would go on to have a lasting effect and also mark the start of a very long journey with my body.

In my early teens, I became sexually active and started using the contraceptive pill (Fig. 2). Things started off well — it really lessened

Figs 1-2

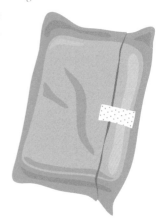

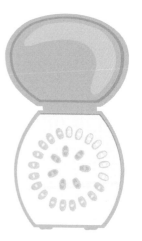

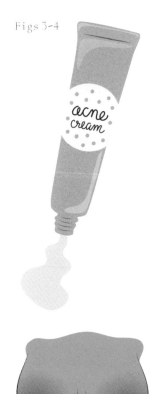

my flow and also reduced pain. It helped my teenage spot-prone skin (Fig. 3) massively, too. However, after a while, the extra hormones I was putting into my body to avoid pregnancy started to mess with me. I would get upset or angry really quickly and wouldn't handle things rationally. I was a pretty moody teenager in any case, and it didn't take long for the pill to send me over the edge. When it started to disagree with me, I would try a different pill. Between the ages of 14 and 20 I must have tried every form available to me. With each pill, different side-effects would arise — suicidal ideation without any explanation, contracting cystitis every time I had sex no matter how careful I was, vaginal dryness, extremely tender boobs (Fig. 4) — you name it, I've experienced it.

I was convinced that my periods would limit me or set me back, and the pill gave me the power to delay or stop them altogether. I would power through the terrible side-effects because I was able to avoid menstruation. Sometimes I would take monthly packets back to back (something my body simply could not handle) if I had a holiday coming up, and eventually just when I couldn't be bothered to have a period. It got to the point where I realized I needed to give my body a break and I'd try to, but I'd inevitably cave every time things got tough. Each month I was met with an overwhelming sense of dread; if I felt even a little bit un-comfortable, I'd jump right back on the pill. Over and over again, unbearable symptoms would all come rushing back, 10 times worse than the month before. There wasn't a day where my boobs didn't ache, my head didn't pound and my vagina didn't feel wrong. It didn't matter that I was suffering, because I wasn't bleeding. It wasn't until I stopped having regular sex that I was able to give my body a break. Yet when I finally gave getting off the pill a proper go, I still couldn't take it. This on-and-off pattern continued and I was stuck in an exhausting cycle for months.

Fig. 5

At the age of 22 it was time to face the music: the pill, no matter what brand, just didn't agree with me. Worried about long-term contraception (birth control) options now that I was in a long-term relationship, I turned to the implant instead. Similarly, it started off great. I was able to have sex with ease and it stopped my periods altogether. It also felt more convenient than taking a pill every day. The fact that this thing in my arm would last for years was very appealing to me, and saying goodbye to my periods was a major plus. The honeymoon period didn't last long, though; the negative side-effects this time were the most awful migraines and bleeding at random points in my cycle (which I soon discovered is referred to as 'spotting'). My doctor suggested taking the pill to counteract this, which was something I wasn't prepared to do.

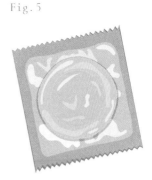

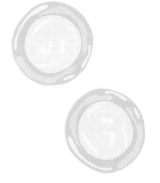

I attempted to ride it out but the symptoms persisted. At one point, spotting turned into bleeding every two weeks. I would be wiped out every other day from migraines on top of this. Once I had exhausted all the options I was willing to try, I came to the conclusion that I didn't want to use any form of hormonal contraception ever again. Enough was enough; condoms (Fig. 5) would suit me just fine. My body quite clearly couldn't handle not having a period, and the most important thing was getting them back. Something had changed within me and made me question everything I'd ever been told about reproductive health. Why does my period have to be this terrible thing every month that I have to put my life on hold for? Why should I put my body through hell to avoid pregnancy when the person I am having sex with can just wear a condom? Am I approaching this all wrong? Does my body need to bleed? How do I resume some form of normalcy? Is that even achievable? I had so many unanswered questions.

After this decision, my body went rogue. The first six months were hell: I would bleed heavily for days on end, I was in so much pain and my hormones were still all over the place. It took near-ly two years for things to work themselves out. My cycle could range anywhere from 18 to 77 days (for comparison, the average cycle length is anywhere between 21 and 35 days). My body was an absolute mess and I found myself almost pining for a regular menstrual cycle. Losing control forced me to reassess the way I viewed my period, and completely changed my attitude towards menstruation in the process.

Although things have improved, I wish I could tell you everything is totally fine now. But the truth is, my uterus and its unusual cycle lengths still bewilder me to this day. I had a good couple of years when my periods would arrive roughly every 29–35 days, but were still heavy and painful. My body eventually fell into a pattern where I'd be regular for three or four months, followed by two cycles in a row when I didn't know whether I was coming or going. Over the course of writing this book, they have only grown more enigmatic. I've seen a handful of doctors (most of whom have been dismissive because I don't exhibit the most common symptoms) and had a range of tests. While I've spoken to hundreds of people who have debilitating periods, I've always put my own menstrual habits down to circumstances like stress or medication. However, I have since been diagnosed with polycystic ovary syndrome (PCOS, which we'll explore in more detail later on; see page 64). The first doctor I saw failed to run all the comprehensive tests, which means I've been liv-ing with this undiagnosed for who knows how long. Frustratingly, this is the case for many people, and is yet another reason I wanted to write this book.

If you're struggling with your periods as you read this, I want to tell you something: *you* know your body better than anyone. If something isn't right, trust yourself, and keep pushing for a different opinion. No periods are the same and this is why it's so important to see a variety of experiences represented equally — now more than ever, since recent studies have found that only one in eight people have a regular 28–day menstrual cycle. Scientists from University College London and femtech app Natural Cycles investigated over 600,000 menstrual cycles (more than 124,000 people) in what is one of the biggest studies of its kind to date. Studying my own body, talking to a range of people and writing this book all helped me realize that reproductive healthcare is all about understanding your own body and what's 'normal' for you.

What made this journey tougher was talking to doctors who lacked empathy, failing to find people going through the same thing and society's general lack of knowledge about periods. I'm someone who finds it hard to deal with things that are out of my control. Confused and completely frustrated with my body, this pushed me to research the hell out of menstruation. I tracked my cycle meticulously (Fig.6), studying the changes in my cervical fluid and making note of any factors that would disrupt my period. I spent a lot of time reading scientific explanations and studies, scouring forums and Facebook groups. I also started to share my findings: I would blog, tweet and talk to my peers about my period and other interesting things I learned along the way. Through this, I found people I could share stories with as well as people who related to me. It seemed so bizarre to me that something so natural, which is often beyond our control, was rarely discussed in a positive way. Who decided that periods are a negative thing and that this is the only way they can be spoken about? If I hadn't decided to stop using certain forms of contraception, I never would have started studying and writing about this topic, which, as it turns out, I am so incredibly passionate about. There is so much I wouldn't be aware of, such as alternative products, other people's experiences, what's happening in other countries, period conditions and the fact that period poos are an actual thing. (Who knew?!)

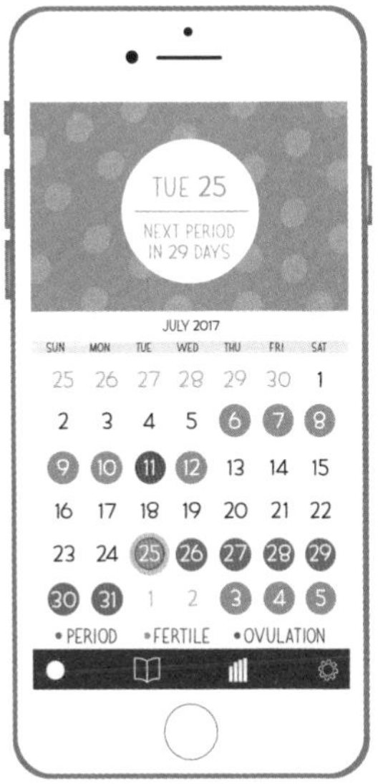

What is *your* relationship with menstruation like? I feel like I let other people's perceptions of periods hinder my own for too long. There's so much out there telling people periods are a shameful thing we can't talk about. Whether it's articles framing normal aspects of menstruation — like simply seeing period blood — as 'gross' (an actual point featured in an article titled 'The 11 Grossest Things Every Woman Does During Her Period' from a 2016 issue of

Fig.6

Cosmopolitan), companies trying to keep menstruation a secret by choosing blue liquid over red in their advertising or refusing to even use the word 'period', or people making you feel ashamed, it's everywhere – and it's bloody exhausting.

Since becoming more vocal about this topic, I've had people write and ask me questions about their bodies: what's normal, why they are experiencing certain symptoms, how to not feel embarrassed. Between harmful myths, a ton of misinformation and a general lack of empathy, it's clear to see that periods are still heavily stigmatized. This outdated way of thinking actively hurts people. It hurts people who have just plucked up the courage to ask for help; it hurts homeless people; it hurts people in developing countries; it hurts transgender and nonbinary people; it hurts those on a lower income. It hurts *everyone* who menstruates. The truth is, menstruation is a natural thing some bodies go through. And for some, a regular cycle is something to be welcomed. Alternatively, a lack of menstruation is also something many are used to. My point is that there is no single universal experience, and language that favours one experience over another can be harmful.

When people *do* talk about menstruation, it's often tailored towards a very specific experience. We usually see a person with a super regular cycle with no other issues present; they also have no problem affording period products. However, this isn't always the case and shouldn't be seen as the default. Over the years, there have been a few books that include other perspectives, such as those written by authors with conditions like endometriosis about their experiences. While these are valid and important, reading about somebody else's experience can sometimes be quite alienating – especially if the author considers that their decisions are the only viable options for anyone else in the same boat. Just because one person decided against surgery in order to manage a condition relating to menstrual health, that doesn't mean everyone in a similar situation has to do so. There isn't just one way that people experience menstruation, and there are so many factors that come into play – and that's okay!

Another thing I think a lot of us do when discussing reproductive health is internalize negative perceptions, which shine

through more than we realize (and many of us, Fig.7
including myself, don't always think about how
our own opinions can affect societal views as a
whole). For a long time I let other people's big
ideas cloud my judgement and it wasn't until
I started speaking to people from all walks of
life that I realized I wasn't alone. With this in
mind, I wanted to write a book (Fig.7) that actively includes people who don't feel seen. The
name *Red Moon Gang* was born years before
I started writing it. Throughout my journey to
understanding my body and raising awareness

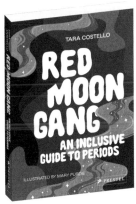

of menstruation, I have always found that periods are one part of
life that can really bring people together. Because so many of us
suffer in silence for so long, it's always incredibly reaffirming when
you meet somebody who doesn't shame you or maybe even experiences something similar to you. Not to mention a massive relief! I
distinctly remember having that feeling after talking to somebody
who just gets it. It's as if you're part of a secret period posse and
there's something empowering about these conversations, even if
they're held privately. Not only did I discover this with two friends,
I also found out we had a mutual appreciation for ridiculous code
names people use for periods, many of which are often, again, so
negative. We joked we were like some sort of pro-period gang, and
that's how the name *Red Moon Gang* came about. Even if it was
just something the three of us used, it's always been in the back of
my mind. It really resonated with me and I wasn't sure why. When
writing this book I wanted to create something that pokes fun at
ridiculous notions and makes people feel less alone. And I think the
title *Red Moon Gang* emulates that perfectly.

The aim of this book is to offer a shame-free and inclusive resource for everyone to enjoy. You don't have to be super in touch with
your cycle (or even have periods); this book will cover everything
from basic anatomy and why people menstruate to alternative menstrual products and how to use them. We'll explore how the way we
talk about periods can sometimes be problematic and discuss the
importance of inclusive language. I want to offer a much-needed

fresh perspective, and hope to inspire you to view menstruation dif—
ferently (even if it's just neutrally). Not everything in this book will
speak directly to you; you can dip in and out, or return to sections as
and when you need to. Take from this book what you need.

Whether you have a period or not, I hope you learn something
and enjoy some of the stories I share along the way. I remember
feeling so alone when trying to navigate my own periods, and I don't
believe anyone should be made to feel like that. The first rule of *Red
Moon Gang*? Make your own rules!

Tara Costello

WHAT A AND IS IMPOR

IS PERIOD WHY IT TANT?

What Happens During a Period

Fig. 8

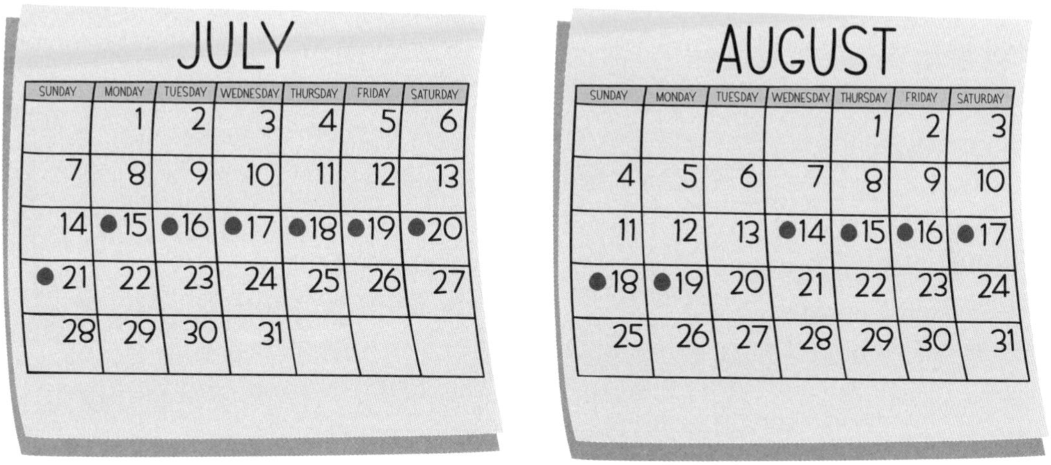

JULY

SUNDAY	MONDAY	TUESDAY	WEDNESDAY	THURSDAY	FRIDAY	SATURDAY
	1	2	3	4	5	6
7	8	9	10	11	12	13
14	●15	●16	●17	●18	●19	●20
●21	22	23	24	25	26	27
28	29	30	31			

AUGUST

SUNDAY	MONDAY	TUESDAY	WEDNESDAY	THURSDAY	FRIDAY	SATURDAY
				1	2	3
4	5	6	7	8	9	10
11	12	13	●14	●15	●16	●17
●18	●19	20	21	22	23	24
25	26	27	28	29	30	31

Periods: that time of the month; the one week out of 30 or so days when blood exits the vagina. A lot of us don't give it much thought beyond the fact that it's just something the body does, particularly if we don't experience it personally. But have you ever stopped and thought about just how *many* people have periods? Think about everyone you interact with on a daily basis, not only people you know. The barista who served you at Starbucks might menstruate, the receptionist you spoke to on the phone, or the person standing next to you in the queue at the post office. A huge proportion of the population menstruates, and this could even include you!

Each month, the body goes through a number of hormone-driven changes to get ready for a possible pregnancy. This series of events is what is known as the menstrual cycle. During each cycle, an egg is developed and released from the ovaries and the lining of the uterus builds up. What does this have to do with a period, you ask? Well, if a pregnancy doesn't happen, the lining sheds during the period and the cycle starts again. This means that a cycle is counted from the first day of one period up to the first day of the next period.

Let's break this down a little, starting with some personal cycle dates straight from my uterus to you (Fig. 8):

Period 1   15–21 July
Period 2   14–19 August
Cycle length   30 days

Although everyone's 'normal' is different, a period that happens every 21 to 35 days is considered a typical regular cycle. Most periods last three to five days on average, but anywhere from two to seven is usual. To calculate my cycle length, I count from 15 July to 13 August. My second period started on 14 August, so this is what I count as day one, which makes it a 30-day cycle. This is what we call period maths! Don't worry if this isn't normal for you; I have personally experienced cycles ranging anywhere from 18 to 77 days over the years. This can occasionally indicate something isn't quite right (more on this later), but sometimes it's just the way our bodies are. Let's try calculating some more cycle lengths:

Period 1   16–20 June
Period 2   15– 21 July
Cycle length   29 days

Period 1   3–9 December
Period 2   15–20 January
Cycle length   43 days

Period 1   25–31 March
Period 2   19–24 May
Cycle length   55 days

To understand the menstrual cycle fully, we need to explore both the reproductive system and the different phases of the cycle in more detail.

Phases of the Menstrual Cycle

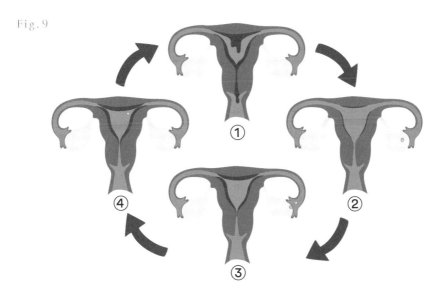

Fig. 9

The entire duration of the menstrual cycle can be divided into four main phases (Fig. 9):

1   Menstrual phase
2   Follicular phase
3   Ovulation phase
4   Luteal phase

The length of a menstrual cycle can differ from person to person, and it can also change over time (my cycles, listed above, are a case in point!). In people who have recently started their periods, the menstrual cycle tends to be longer, and it can get shorter with age. Ultimately, it's the rise and fall of hormone levels that control the cycle and eventually trigger a period. Two hormones you are going to see mentioned a lot throughout this book are oestrogen and progesterone. This pair have a number of effects on the body but, during the menstrual cycle in particular, oestrogen is mainly involved in building up the lining of the uterus, while progester-one focuses on maintaining the lining in preparation for pregnancy. Here's exactly what happens to the body through each stage of the menstrual cycle.

① MENSTRUAL PHASE

The menstrual phase starts when an egg from the previous cycle isn't fertilized. When pregnancy doesn't take place, hormone levels start to drop. As the uterine lining that has thickened over the course of the cycle is no longer needed, it has to shed. During the period the uterine lining — along with blood, cells and other fluid — sheds by exiting the vagina. In the simplest terms, menstruation, or having a period, is the body's way of releasing tissue it no longer needs (thank u, next!).

Periods usually start anywhere between the ages of 10 and 15, with the average age thought to be around 12. It can also start earlier or later, as everyone develops at different rates. While there is no wrong or right age to start having periods, a visit to the doctor is advised if they haven't started by the age of 16. And if you're wondering how much bloodshed to expect, 5 to 80 ml of blood (or, up to five tablespoons) is thought to be the average amount lost each period. Anything above 80 ml is considered heavy menstrual bleeding. It's easy to overestimate, as it can look and feel like a lot more sometimes.

You may be thinking, 'What do I do with this information? Do I need to be measuring my blood — and how the hell do I do that?' The general rule of thumb is to talk to a doctor if a period is affecting your daily life or lasting longer than a week, or if you're going through a high volume of products a day. For reference, changing every hour shouldn't be ignored. If you want to be more aware, then using a menstrual cup is probably the easiest way to monitor the menstrual flow yourself. For example, one brand I use (Mooncup) is 46 mm (1.2 in.) in diameter and I've only ever filled it to the top a handful of times. Don't worry, we'll get to the wonder that is reusable menstrual products all in good time (see pages 88–93).

So now, let's talk period blood. It can come in a wide variety of consistencies. I did not realize how thick mine was until I started using a menstrual cup. Our flows can be heavy, light, somewhere in between, or change at different points. For example, mine is like the lift scene from *The Shining* for about two to three days, then I'm pretty light afterwards. I've also experienced periods where my flow is light for a day and then suddenly returns to absolute chaos.

Fig. 10

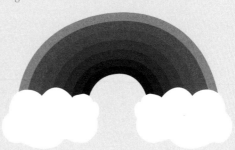

The same can be said for colours: over the years I've seen a range of red hues exit my body, as well as brown period blood. Different colours can mean different things. Bright red blood means the uterine lining is shedding at a steady rate, as this is the freshest blood. Did you know that the longer blood has been in the uterus, the darker it becomes? Dark red blood is likely to show up first thing in the morning or when your period is heavier than usual. This particular shade of red can also indicate that the shedding is beginning to slow down, which is why blood can appear darker towards the end of a period. Brown menstrual blood is also associated with blood shedding at a slower rate; it can make an appearance at the beginning of the period (sometimes left over from last month. No, really!) or right at the end. Consider this a menstrual rainbow (Fig. 10) of sorts!

It is also perfectly normal for blood to appear clumpy from time to time; finding blood clots on toilet paper is a reality for many of us, particularly when the flow is dark and heavy. Blood clots are just tissue that cannot be broken down, however; if they are bigger than the size of a large coin, they should be investigated. Sometimes blood can be extremely light red or almost pink when a period is lighter than usual, or when a person is spotting (light vaginal bleeding that happens just before or outside of regular periods). Orange or rust-coloured blood and dark blood with a blue/purple hue to it are shades that might indicate something is wrong, especially if the consistency, texture and/or scent feel off as well, and you should get this looked into.

The menstrual cycle does not always run like clockwork: sometimes it can be irregular. What does this mean? Well, they say a typical menstrual cycle should last around 22–35 days. Menstrual bleeding is considered irregular if cycles are outside of the range 21–45 days (adolescents) or 24–38 days (adults), or if cycles vary in length by more than seven to nine days (for example, a cycle that is 27 days long one month, followed by 42 the next) and last longer than eight days. People with irregular cycles may notice their period turns up early, shows up late or even skips the party altogether. To determine whether your cycle is irregular, count from the last day of your previous period and stop counting on the first day of your next. If the gap between your periods starting keeps changing, like mine, you probably have an irregular cycle. While this can sometimes be the first sign something is not quite right, it's not *always* a big deal. Whether it's due to hormone imbalance, stress, medication or other illnesses, people experience irregular periods more than you think. After 15 years of menstruating, I'm pretty sure I've had more irregular cycles than regular at this point. If you're concerned, consult your doctor. They may suggest some form of hormonal contraception, but remember this isn't your only option if you'd like to avoid that route.

Changes in the body's hormone levels before a period can cause physical and emotional changes, and these are commonly referred to as premenstrual syndrome (PMS). Symptoms such as cramps, tender breasts, bloating, mood swings, irritability, headaches, tiredness and low back pain can be experienced during this time. What fascinates me most about periods is that everyone's 'normal' can differ wildly. My period, and the symptoms that come with it, can change at any given time for a number of reasons, whereas some people have a pretty similar experience each time. One thing that never changes for me is the fact that day two of my period is without fail the worst day of my entire cycle every month.

② FOLLICULAR PHASE

Is that enough period talk for you? Just kidding, there's loads more to come! Let's move onto the next phase, which is known as the follicular phase. This starts on the first day of the period and lasts until ovulation. Follicle stimulating hormone (FSH) is a hormone that stimulates the egg cells in the ovaries to grow. At the beginning of each cycle, the pituitary gland (a tiny organ the size of a pea found within the base of the brain) secretes FSH and encourages the ovaries to produce mature eggs. Each egg grows in its own individual, fluid-filled sac called a follicle. The FSH stimulates a number of follicles to develop and start producing oestrogen. The levels of oestrogen are at their lowest on the first day of the period, but from here on out they start to increase as the follicles grow. As the follicles develop, they produce oestrogen.

As this stage of the menstrual cycle progresses, the heat is on. Rising up like the next Supreme, one dominant egg matures within the enlarging follicle and suppresses the rest. While this is happening, the increasing amount of oestrogen works on thickening the uterine lining. As I said earlier, even if you have no intention of getting pregnant, the body still functions as if you're going to change your mind and continues with these preparations. You know, just in case. Once the dominant egg is released at ovulation, the empty follicle that is left in the ovary (which is called the corpus luteum) is what releases progesterone (in a higher amount) and oestrogen (in a lower amount). Together, these hormones make sure the uterus is thick with nutrients and blood on the off chance a fertilized egg would have all it needs to grow (Fig. 11). If the released egg isn't fertilized, the corpus luteum breaks down, causing the secretion of both these hormones to stop (this is what triggers the lining of the uterus to exit the body). Once ovulation has been and gone, the rest of the follicles should reabsorb into the body, but in many cases (such as in people with PCOS) this doesn't always happen.

Fig. 11

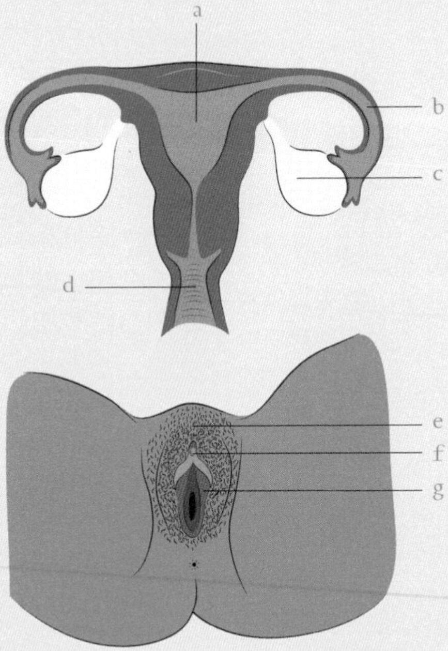

a Uterus
b Fallopian tubes
c Ovaries
d Vagina
e Mons pubis
f Clitoris
g Labia

The average follicular phase is 16 days, but it can last anywhere from 11 to 27 days depending on cycle length. The length of the follicular phase depends in part on the amount of time it takes our dominant follicle to rise through the ranks and come into its power.

③ OVULATION PHASE

Ovulation: the part of the menstrual cycle we see play out most frequently onscreen. You know, when characters in a film who are trying to get pregnant get upset about missing the opportunity to have sex at the right time and become frustrated by having to wait an entire month before trying again? But what we don't often see depicted is how this actually works.

As the level of oestrogen is still increasing, it eventually triggers a surge in luteinizing hormone (an LH surge). This hormone causes the dominant follicle to rupture and release the mature egg. From here it travels to the Fallopian tube. This process is known as ovulation. This is an important part of the cycle for those wanting to have a baby; you simply cannot conceive without ovulating. In each cycle there is a 'fertile window': this is the day an egg is released (ovulation) and the days in the run-up to it. The window depends on the length of the menstrual cycle and can vary. The core concept of trying to get pregnant involves scheduling sex during this particular part of the cycle. Sperm can live for up to five days in the body, so having sex during the fertile window allows the best chance of getting pregnant (Fig. 12). While the fertile window can take place over almost a week, ovulation happens over a mere 24 hours. This explains people's frustration — you have only one day to fertilize the egg.

Fig. 12

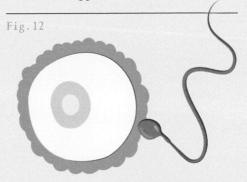

Birth control, such as the contraceptive pill, prevents ovulation by maintaining more consistent hormone levels. Without a peak in oestrogen, the ovary doesn't get the signal to release an egg. The pill in particular also thickens cervical mucus so that sperm cannot infiltrate. Emergency contraception like the 'morning after' pill does the same, and also works to prevent the union of the sperm and egg. If fertilization has already occurred, it may prevent the egg from attaching to the uterus (implantation). However, if a fertilized egg has implanted prior to taking emergency contraception, it will not work. There's a reason it's called the 'morning after' pill and not the 'week after'!

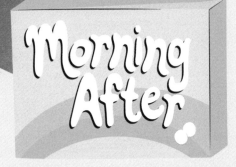

Are there any signs of ovulation to look out for? Yes, absolutely! The three main signs that can be studied to predict ovulation are changes in basal body temperature (BBT), the position and firmness of the cervix and cervical fluid. You can also use ovulation predictor kits (OPKs) to detect a surge in the production of luteinizing hormone (LH). That's right: in addition to blood and tissue, cervical mucus (or fluid) is another thing that exits the body and can change throughout the menstrual cycle.

WHAT'S THAT IN MY UNDERWEAR?

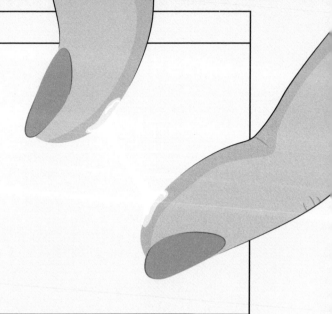

WHAT IS IT?

Cervical mucus is a fluid secreted by the cervix and is stimulated by the hormone oestrogen. It's most commonly referred to as cervical fluid, cervical discharge or vaginal discharge. In fact, there is somewhat of a debate happening right now surrounding the term 'vaginal discharge'. Some feel the word 'discharge' has negative connotations and makes people perceive this fluid as something that should be given no second thought when, really, it's very important. The scientific term is in fact 'cervical mucus', but there is something about the word 'mucus' that makes people run for the hills — perhaps because we associate it with the alarmingly coloured stuff that comes out of your nose when you're ill.

Recently, there has been a rise in people taking back the real scientific term. In the interest of destigmatizing, I will be referring to it as cervical mucus. However, I do personally use both 'mucus' and 'fluid' interchangeably, and there are of course times where I'll refer to it as 'that goopy stuff you find in your underwear' when talking to somebody who is unfamiliar with it. Call it whatever you feel comfortable with!

WHAT DOES IT DO?

It carries away dead cells and bacteria that in turn keep the vagina clean (similar to how saliva cleanses the mouth) and helps prevent infection. It can also signify when a person is fertile, or when something is wrong. Think of cervical mucus as the vagina's method of housekeeping.

WHAT DOES IT LOOK LIKE?

Cervical mucus can often appear clear, cloudy-white and/or yellowish. It can be thick and stringy at different points in the menstrual cycle, too. It changes in appearance, texture and amount throughout the month based on oestrogen levels. Changes in mucus can occur for a number of different reasons, such as emotional stress, nutritional status, pregnancy, sexual arousal and even usage of certain medications.

WHEN DOES IT TYPICALLY OCCUR THROUGHOUT THE CYCLE?

- Before a period: It is normal to have some dry days leading up to a period.
- During a period: Blood flow makes it difficult to see cervical mucus, but it's there.
- The day after a period: This is typically when the least amount of cervical mucus is produced and the chances of getting pregnant are lowest. In fact, some people report feeling quite dry or not seeing much fluid at all during this point in the cycle.
- The week after a period: Thin mucus with a light white colour may start to make an appearance around this time and your underwear may feel a little damp. However, this type of mucus still signifies low fertility.
- When ovulation may be coming: Thicker mucus that has a creamy appearance or feels sticky indicates you are going into your most fertile stage of the cycle.
- When ovulation is very close: Cervical mucus becomes thinner and more watery.
- As you approach ovulation: Oestrogen levels begin to surge, triggering the cervix to secrete cervical mucus of fertile quality. This type of mucus is clear, stretchy and often referred to as egg white cervical mucus (EWCM).
- After ovulation: In the days leading up to your period, there may be less mucus being produced and it may appear cloudy and sticky.
- After implantation: You may notice a heavier flow of mucus.
- During pregnancy: Increased mucus is expected as the delivery date nears. The cervix begins to dilate and releases thick (clear or blood-streaked) mucus, also referred to as 'the mucus plug'.

I'd also like to note that thick, slightly yellow mucus without a smell is quite normal. It can be a clue a period is coming or a sign of early pregnancy.

These are general types to look out for, but of course everybody is different. If you are looking to understand your cycle better and want to pinpoint exactly when you ovulate, tracking your menstrual cycle and cervical mucus is a great idea. There are a number of websites or even fertility coaches out there who provide insight and material on fertility charting (head to page 167 for a list of recommendations).

WHEN SHOULD I SEE A DOCTOR?

If your cervical mucus has a strong odour that seems 'off' or it appears overly thick, you might require a visit to the doctor. Colours that are a cause for concern include green, pink and grey shades. Cervical mucus that is clumpy and resembles cottage cheese (perhaps not the most pleasant mental image, but I guarantee you know exactly what I mean) should definitely be investigated. Cervical mucus that is accompanied by other symptoms, such as itching, rashes, soreness or pain during urination, shouldn't be ignored either.

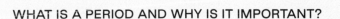

Your body produces more cervical mucus before an egg is released. Just before ovulation, as oestrogen levels rise (Fig. 13), you may see an influx of clear, watery mucus. This slippery mucus reminiscent of egg whites is often referred to as 'egg white cervical mucus' (EWCM). It has a stretchy consistency and may appear yellow, white or cloudy. EWCM is 'sperm-friendly': it allows sperm to swim through more easily and survive. The appearance of EWCM is a sign that ovulation is about to occur, and having this type of mucus during your fertile window improves your chances of conceiving.

As I've become older, cervical mucus has become something that really intrigues me. It can offer a person so much insight into their cycle and yet it's been completely demonized. I remember when I was younger feeling absolutely horrified when I found orange and white stains in my knickers, scared that something was seriously wrong with my body. I was so scared, in fact, that I didn't tell anybody and just carried on as normal. I didn't learn until years later that vaginal fluid is acidic by nature and as a result can 'bleach' your underwear. Thankfully nothing was wrong, but

can you imagine if it was? I would have done nothing because I felt too ashamed to ask anyone if it was normal or not. If cervical mucus is a nuisance and ruining too much of your underwear, try wearing panty liners. Who says you can't use these products outside your period? (Reusable cloth panty liners exist if disposables aren't your thing, or if you can't afford to keep buying them.)

What's fun about having a healthy relationship with your bodily functions is the thrill when you correctly guess where you are in your menstrual cycle. A little game I like to play whenever I spot a noticeable change in cervical mucus is to check my period app and see how far off I am. I still haven't quite figured out what day ovulation takes place, but I do a little cheer every time I guess my fertile window right. And if you try this and you're still none the wiser, never fear! Just keep studying your body and you'll soon become acquainted. There are wonderful resources out there that can help you chart your cycle (again, head to page 167). After years of not knowing what my body was up to, it feels good and somewhat empowering to have a better understanding.

Fig. 13

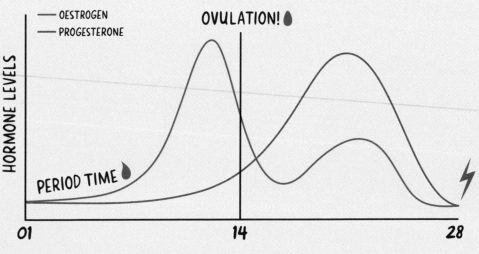

HORMONE CHANGES IN AN AVERAGE CYCLE

Fig. 14

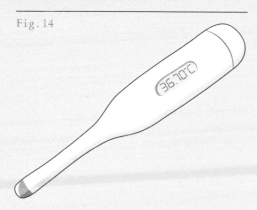

Another way to predict ovulation is by tracking your basal body temperature (BBT) (Fig. 14), the lowest body temperature attained during rest (normally during sleep). Many healthcare professionals recommend measuring BBT immediately after waking up or before any physical activity has happened for the most accurate reading. As ovulation looms closer there may be a slight decline, but it will be followed by a sharp increase soon after; the increase in BBT is another sign ovulation has just happened. BBT rises after ovulation thanks to increased progesterone released from the corpus luteum, and it stays high if a pregnancy has occurred. It tends to stay in the higher range throughout the luteal (post-ovulation) phase until the next cycle begins. At the end of the luteal phase your temperature will drop and your period should follow. Noticing the drop in temperature at the end of the luteal phase is how some people get an idea their period is due to arrive!

Like cervical mucus and BBT, the cervix also goes through changes during the cycle. Typically around ovulation it can be described as open, soft and very high. For good measure, here's how the cervix changes throughout the menstrual cycle (as well as during pregnancy):

- During menstrual bleeding: The cervix is typically lower than normal, opening slightly to allow blood to flow out, and feels hard — like the tip of the nose!

- After a period ends: The cervix remains low and hard while the opening to the uterus remains closed.

- At the height of ovulation: During this time, the cervix feels more like the inside of your cheek as the uterus is open to allow sperm to enter. Sometimes the cervix becomes so soft that it blends in with the vaginal walls, rising so high that a finger cannot reach it.

- Once ovulation occurs: The cervix eventually drops and becomes more firm (like the tip of a nose again). The opening to the uterus becomes tightly closed, which sometimes happens immediately after ovulation but can take hours, or even days.

- When pregnancy occurs: The cervix will rise up and become soft, but still remains tightly closed. This can happen at different times for different people, sometimes as early as 12 days after ovulation or after the pregnancy has been confirmed.

- During pregnancy: Throughout pregnancy, the cervix will gradually soften as the body gets ready for labour. The cervix will decrease in length and become thinner before finally opening in order to prepare for giving birth.

When the body's level of luteinizing hormone rises, it triggers the start of ovulation. The LH surge begins around 36 hours before ovulation and, as we've covered already, once the egg is released it only survives for about 24 hours. So if you're trying to conceive, noting the timing of the LH surge can help. OPKs contain at-home tests that measure LH levels in urine; you can buy them without a prescription from health and beauty stores or online. A positive result means that a person has a high amount of LH in their system. Levels drop after ovulation, so the tests should only show positive results during fertile times. The idea is to start testing levels when the fertile window is drawing near. However, there are a few disadvantages, and OPKs may not be the right choice for everyone. For example, if a person has irregular cycles, testing can be unreliable, expensive and frustrating all-round. People with PCOS may experience persistently high LH levels (and tests many even show positive results throughout their cycles), as might those who are approaching menopause, which can make results unreliable. Testing at the right time is essential, and that's why it's recommended that you track a combination of the things listed above to try and figure out when you're ovulating.

In my experience, another lesser-known side-effect of ovulation is pain in the lower abdomen. Sometimes the cramps I experience when I'm ovulating are more painful than period pain! I've also heard people say they experience ovulation pain on the side of whichever ovary is producing eggs. Other reported signs that ovulation is due are a heightened sense of smell, breast soreness or tenderness, light spotting or brown fluid and a heightened sex drive.

Ovulation typically takes place between days 10 and 19 of the cycle, roughly 12 to 16 days before the next period. So it is usually assumed to occur in the middle of your cycle, but like everything else it can vary from cycle to cycle.

④ LUTEAL PHASE

We're at the final stage of the menstrual cycle now; we made it! The luteal phase starts on the day of ovulation and ends when the next period begins. After an egg is released, it moves into the Fallopian tube and stays there waiting for a single sperm to fertilize it. As we've mentioned, the egg can only be fertilized for 24 hours. So, what happens if conception is successful? If the egg and sperm meet, they join and the sperm fertilizes the egg. When the egg reaches the uterus, it attaches itself to the uterine lining and pregnancy will begin.

A fertilized egg that becomes implanted in the uterus will develop an embryo and placenta, and eventually a baby grows. That is how a baby is made, kids! There are some exceptions worth mentioning here, such as the case of twins. Identical twins occur when one fertilized egg splits into two separate cells; the same can be said for identical triplets, quads and higher multiples as well. Non-identical twins occur when two eggs are released and fertilized separately. But, if no sperm is around to fertilize the egg, it simply moves through the uterus and disintegrates.

Whether fertilization takes place or not, the follicle still releases an egg. Once the mature egg is released, the follicle closes and forms a hormone-secreting structure (the corpus luteum), which produces increasing quantities of progesterone. Remember I mentioned this hormone at the beginning of the chapter? I bet you were wondering when it would show up! Well, here's where it gets to shine: progesterone helps the uterus prepare for the implantation of a developing embryo. If a fertilized egg implants in the uterus, it sends signals to the ovary to keep making this precious hormone, as it makes the uterine lining thick and nourishing to help sustain a pregnancy. If a pregnancy does happen, the body will also produce human chorionic gonadotropin (hCG), a hormone that some pregnancy tests detect. This aids in maintaining the corpus luteum, as well as helping the uterine lining get thicker. If a pregnancy doesn't occur, the corpus luteum will shrink and reabsorb into the body. This, in turn, leads to decreased levels of both oestrogen and progesterone, which triggers menstruation (Fig. 15) and brings us full circle.

A luteal phase typically lasts anywhere from 11 to 17 days, with the average length being 14 days. Symptoms of premenstrual syndrome (PMS) such as bloating, breast pain, food cravings, changes in sexual desire and mood and headaches can be experienced during this time, in case you ever thought you were experiencing PMS super early. Since a short luteal phase is associated with difficulty conceiving and early pregnancy loss, most people don't pay attention to it unless they are having trouble getting pregnant. To calculate the luteal phase length, count the number of days between ovulation and the start of the next period. Experts say you ideally want 12 or more days, and anything under 10 is considered short. Thus, a person has a short luteal phase if they get their period 10 days or fewer after they ovulate.

To recap: several follicles grow each cycle, with only one reaching its final form and releasing a mature egg. If the egg doesn't become fertilized it reabsorbs into the body, and then the lining of the uterus breaks down and sheds out of the vagina during the period. This process is repeated every month until the menopause (typically starting from age 45 onwards), which is when periods end and a person is no longer able to get pregnant naturally. I understand this is a lot of information to take in but don't worry, there won't be a quiz at the end of the chapter. Hold onto this book and return to it whenever you need a refresher, or to educate someone else.

Fig. 15

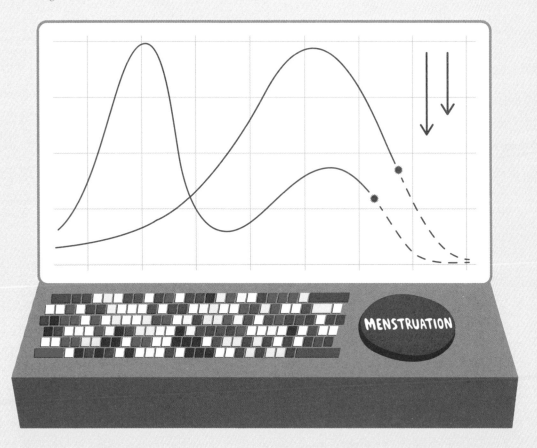

Is All This *Really* Important?

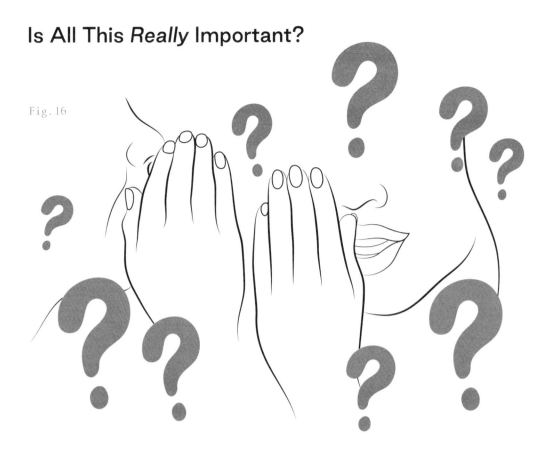

Fig. 16

The answer is yes! Hear me out. What you've just read is how an average cycle generally works and how a period without any other issues flows, but it's not always this black and white (or red). There are a wild amount of factors that can affect the menstrual cycle, with some still being discovered. Sudden changes in menstruation (or the vagina in general) can sometimes reveal a lot about what's going on with a person, be it physical or emotional. For example, experiencing 50- to 88-day-long cycles allowed me to gain better insight into my mental state and forced me to re-evaluate certain aspects of my life. I experienced these unorthodox (for me) cycle lengths for a good part of a year, and I didn't even realize how stressed I was until a doctor spelled it out for me.

Irregular cycles can also be an indication of more serious health issues such as an overactive thyroid, fibroids or conditions like poly-cystic ovary syndrome (PCOS). The same can be said for extremely bad period pain; although pain is common, it shouldn't be debilitating.

Often it's one of the first signs that something isn't quite right, as it can indicate serious conditions such as uterine cysts or endometriosis (where tissue similar to the endometrial tissue that lines the uterus grows in other places, such as on the ovaries or Fallopian tubes). Changes in both menstrual flow / patterns and cervical mucus can also reveal important information regarding overall health. Things like whether or not a pregnancy has occurred, how a person reacts to certain medication, nutritional status or if there's a deficiency somewhere are just a few examples of issues that these changes could be hinting at. A change in mucus is also one of the first noticeable signs of a sexually transmitted disease (STD).

Absence of menstruation can indicate a few things too, particularly for those trying to figure out whether they're pregnant or not. It makes sense if you think about all the other ways bodies show us something is wrong, like getting a headache if you've been staring at a screen too long or questionable bowel movements when you've eaten something that doesn't agree with you. The appearance, frequency and consistency of menstrual blood and certain symptoms can provide invaluable information. Whether it's a benign issue or something a little more serious, these things are clues. Which makes you question the phrase 'it's just a period', doesn't it?

So, why isn't any of this information considered common knowledge? Why do so many people either inadvertently persevere through pain or get forced to downplay and ignore their body's signals? I'll tell you why: there's a stigma surrounding menstruation that has been securely in place for centuries. Long-held societal taboos are often pre-agricultural, and are still subtly reinforced every day. The way people feel the need to lower their voices when discussing their periods (Fig. 16) or hide the products they're using, brands choosing blue liquid over red in their adverts: these are just a few small examples of behaviour that perpetuates the idea that a period is something that shouldn't be discussed openly. This might not sound like a big deal, but together these instances add up and contribute to a much larger issue. Years of entertaining the idea that a period needs to be hidden has led to a lack of knowledge and understanding about reproductive health, as well as widespread dismissal of what are tediously referred to as 'women's issues'. In reality, this unnecessary gendering of the language surrounding reproductive health only alienates people, particularly transgender and nonbinary people.

The truth is, most people (even if they don't menstruate) probably can't pinpoint the exact moment they came to feel so negatively towards periods. However, the problem is that they *do* — and many don't think to question it. I mean, I get it. When we absorb harmful societal beliefs from every direction, it's almost impossible not to be affected by them in some way. If most people around you agree, why would you challenge the status quo? But, here's the thing: the effects are universal and cause varying levels of damage across the globe. The fallout of these attitudes and long-held customs take years to unravel and we're still picking up the pieces now. The longer this feeling of shame is alive, the longer people will continue to be kept in the dark. Since shame categorically stops people from seeking help, talking about periods is a vital step in working towards eradicating practices that alienate and hurt people. Real change comes from challenging stigma and dismantling it, and every avalanche starts with just one snowflake (Fig. 17).

We as a society are slowly chipping away at the unfair lens through which menstruation has been viewed. In recent years, there has been a rise in people who are starting to challenge these narrow views and unfair attitudes, and who instead encourage visibility and inclusion. Many are calling to take back control of their bodies after years of being told using hormonal contraception was their only choice, and are pushing for more answers while menstruating again. A variety of people experience menstruation and, I don't know about you, but I'm tired of all the inaccuracies, lack of representation beyond the average experience, language that discourages people and shameful attitudes that are impossible to escape when trying to find resources and help. The truth is that periods matter and it's about time we started acting like it. Let us debunk and demystify this natural bodily function once and for all!

Fig. 17

What Do You Call Your Period?

Checking into the Red Roof Inn

The Painters and Decorators Are In

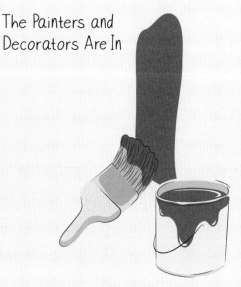

Visitor from Hell

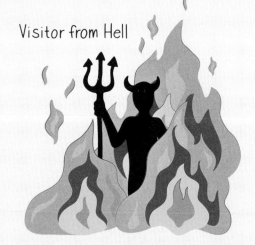

The Red Badge of Courage

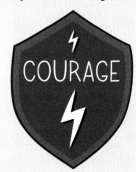

Rebooting the Ovarian Operating System

Shark Week

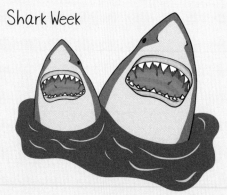

The Red Wedding

Surfing the Crimson Wave

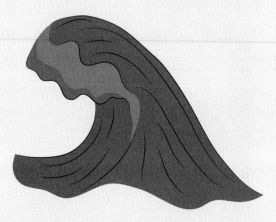

Riding the Cotton Pony

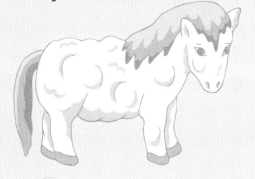

A Visit from Aunt Flo

WHAT

WHEN

YOU'RE

TO EXPECT

PMSING

Blame It on the Hormones

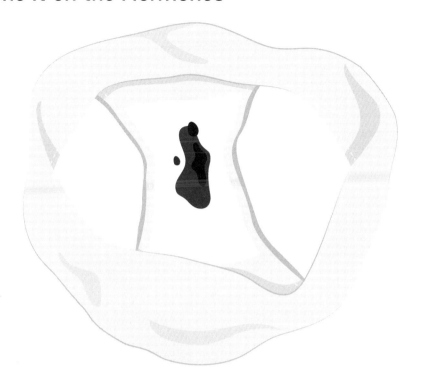

Crying for no apparent reason? Missed your stop on the bus? Accidentally dropped your phone? Hulking out over something trivial? Trapped wind? Blame it on the hormones, babe, it kind of helps.

As if dealing with the sheer volume of fluid that can exit one's body during a period isn't stressful enough, there's a ton of symptoms that come with it too. You may have heard people complain about PMS in passing — or, if you're like me, you just wail, 'I'm PMSing!' at anyone who will listen. It stands for premenstrual syndrome, which refers to symptoms experienced before a period starts. They're a barrel of laughs, I can assure you. It's also commonly referred to as PMT, which stands for premenstrual tension. These symptoms can be physical, mental and sometimes even behavioural. The most commonly discussed symptoms of PMS are feeling bloated, stomach cramps, backaches, sore breasts, breaking out, nausea, food cravings and mood swings. Most onscreen representations of PMS will depict somebody feeling upset, emotional, irritable or angry (sometimes all at once, which to be fair is often an accurate depiction of me when I'm PMSing).

Fig. 18

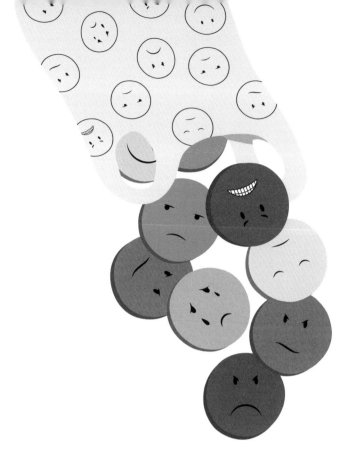

PMS can start as early as two weeks leading up to a period, but again, some bodies have different ideas. I myself seem to
go through a rather tedious pattern. I'll have a couple of somewhat
manageable and light periods where I experience PMS for only a
few days beforehand and sometimes up until the beginning of my
period, followed by one that is complete anarchy. All hell breaks
loose around 10 days before my period, when I experience a not-
so-festive countdown; it's blood, sweat, irrational anger and tears
from start to finish.

Right off the bat, I'm going to say that if you've ever felt that
the emotions you go through in the run-up to a period (as well as
the speed and intensity at which you fly through them without a
moment's notice) make you feel like a ridiculous, irrational person —
I promise, you're not alone. As somebody who suffers greatly and
often finds themselves on a PMS warpath, I feel you. It's not all
in your head. I mean, yes, there are probably times where you've

overreacted, but let me be facetious for a moment, okay? The strug-gle is real! Besides, you could react badly to something on *any* day of your cycle; your patience just happens to be pretty thin when blood is exiting your body at a rapid speed! Trust me, your feelings are definitely valid. Anyone who tries to suggest otherwise will auto-matically be subjected to a rant. Sorry, I don't make the rules.

So, what causes PMS? Like many things relating to reproductive health, the exact cause of PMS isn't fully understood and has not yet been scientifically proven. However, it is strongly suggested that it's due to changes in hormone levels during the menstrual cycle. If you revert back to the previous chapter where the cycle is explained in more detail, this does make sense, considering how hormones are constantly changing. Whether it's an influx of oestrogen or low pro-gesterone (or perhaps a combination of the two), it's bound to have some sort of effect on you.

Sometimes hormone levels change only slightly, which could explain why you're a raging bag of emotions (Fig. 18) while your friend is barely suffering. It's like everything else (such as pain threshold, tastes and allergic reactions) — our bodies have their own unique ways of reacting to changes we go through. As this book progresses, you'll see we're all about the lesser-discussed parts of menstruation here. Chances are, if you've experienced something that happens around your period that you thought wasn't just coincidental, you might find a reason for it. If not, just comfort me, okay? Please. Let's get a PMS support group going; we can all cry together. As hormone changes are thought to be the biggest contributing factor, it's a time when I blame absolutely everything and anything on them. I'm giving you permission to do so too, and if you've been menstruating for a while now, I think you've more than earned the right!

Let's explore this hormone theory a little more. In case you weren't aware, hormones are an extremely complicated (fun!) sys-tem in the human body. They're responsible for a ton of things that affect our everyday lives, such as sleeping patterns, weight fluctu-ations, growth and development and, of course, our moods. They should rise and fall fluidly but they're in an incredibly delicate balance, so it doesn't always work out that way. Ideally you want your body to cycle through its functions without difficulty, and hormones play a key part in that. Let's circle back to our all-important duo oestrogen and progesterone; think of them as the yin and yang of your cycle. Oestrogen is the active yang, while progesterone is the yin that grounds us. Too much yang without yin to balance us out can cause issues: for example, elevated levels of oestrogen have been linked to anxiety. This could also explain why so many people find the contraceptive pill makes their mood change, as they are essentially pumping more hormones into their bodies.

People who already suffer with their mental health may find PMS hits them particularly hard, as chemical levels in the brain can fluctuate during this time as well. One that fluctuates in particular is serotonin (Fig. 19), a chemical known to help balance and regulate moods that make you feel happier. When oestrogen starts to drop, serotonin can too; people with mental illnesses that stem from low serotonin levels (depression, anxiety and OCD, to name a few) are likely to find the unpleasant symptoms of PMS more disruptive. As somebody who suffers with both anxiety and depression, I know my PMS symptoms are definitely worse when I'm going through a bad time mentally. Despite this, nobody seems to really talk about the extent to which PMS can affect you emotionally. Sometimes, I find it near impossible to function; I become completely tongue-tied and forget things. I can be in the middle of talking and completely lose my train of thought or add in a nonsensical word. Often, self-doubt will wash over me and I'll find it hard to focus.

I wanted to find out if others feel overwhelmed in the run-up to their period, as I do. I spoke to a range of people while writing this book, and it has been comforting to find that many of them experience this frustration and self-doubt too. It can be a very isolating time for many of us and no matter how familiar you are with menstruating, it doesn't always get easier. Of all the ways unbalanced hormones affect me, one of the most annoying symptoms has to be my heightened emotions and more sensitive state. I'm a water sign (Cancer, represent!), so I'm pretty emotional on any given day, but in the run-up to my period it reaches new heights. Everything generally hits me a lot harder; the tiniest and most insignificant thing can set me off. Joking about this element of PMS or a particularly fragile mental state can bring comfort, of course, but sometimes these situations can also be really tough to navigate, especially when you've got to get on with things!

One person I spoke to told me about a time when her emotions were more upsetting than amusing: 'I really wanted a can of Pepsi, so I went to the shop but found it was closed. Naturally, I spent 20 minutes crying in bed about it. Sounds funny and ridiculous, but it's actually horrible having no control over your emotions and feeling like you've ruined your weekend.' This is something many of us can relate to. A lot of people don't take mental health seriously enough as it is — whether it's observing our own mental state or considering the wellbeing of others — but it's high time we did.

Fig. 19

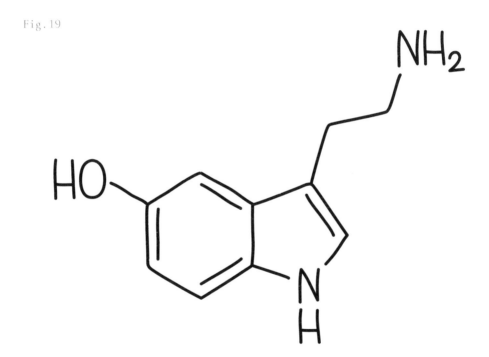

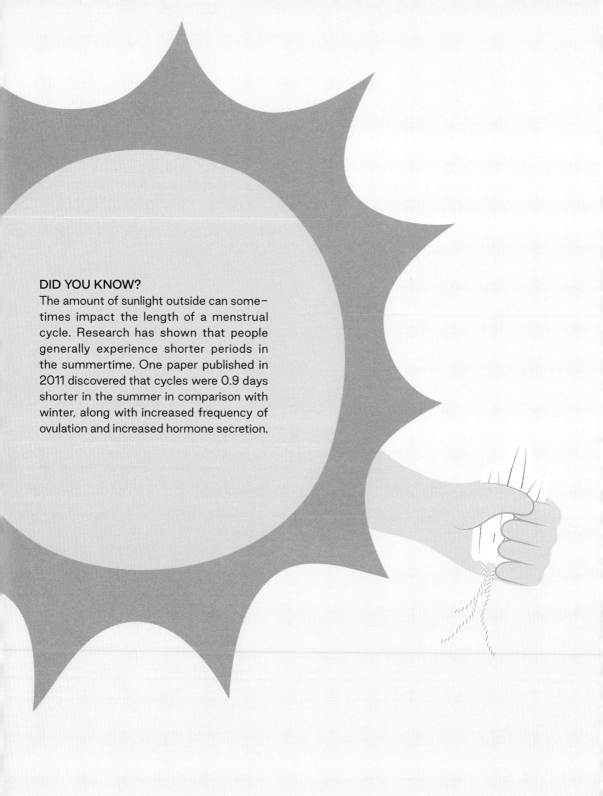

DID YOU KNOW?
The amount of sunlight outside can sometimes impact the length of a menstrual
cycle. Research has shown that people
generally experience shorter periods in
the summertime. One paper published in
2011 discovered that cycles were 0.9 days
shorter in the summer in comparison with
winter, along with increased frequency of
ovulation and increased hormone secretion.

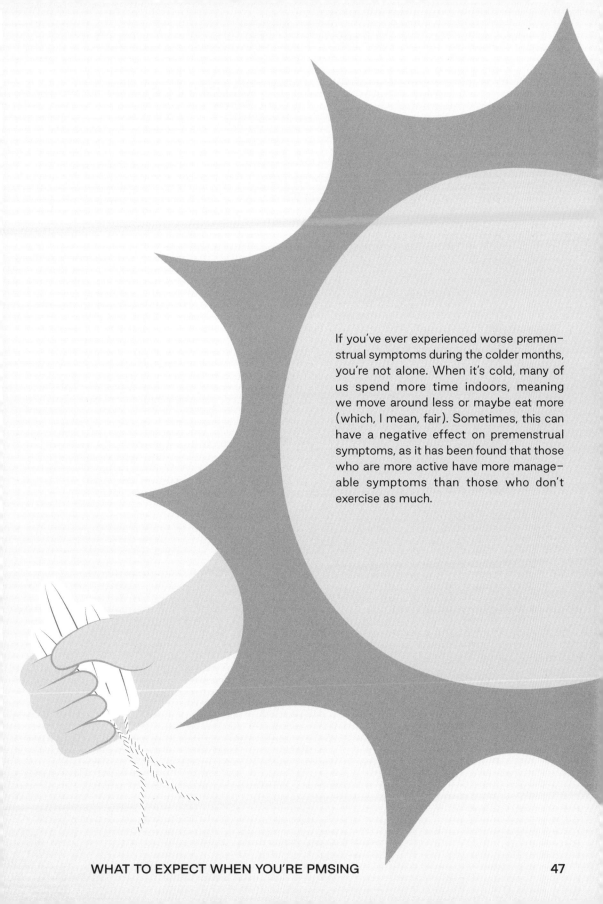

If you've ever experienced worse premen-strual symptoms during the colder months, you're not alone. When it's cold, many of us spend more time indoors, meaning we move around less or maybe eat more (which, I mean, fair). Sometimes, this can have a negative effect on premenstrual symptoms, as it has been found that those who are more active have more manage-able symptoms than those who don't exercise as much.

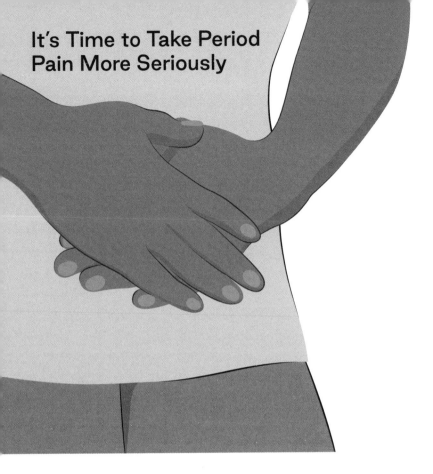

It's Time to Take Period Pain More Seriously

Period pain in particular should never be ignored, especially since there is now more evidence than ever that proves just how serious it can be. In 2016, John Guillebaud, Emeritus Professor of Family Planning and Reproductive Health at University College London, revealed that research suggests period pain can be 'almost as bad as having a heart attack'. (I mean, not hard to believe, right? Anyone who menstruates could tell you how bad it can be!) He believed the reason it hadn't been given the centrality it should have was partly because cisgender (those whose sense of personal identity and gender match the sex they were assigned at birth) men don't experience or understand it. Obviously not all doctors are cisgender men, but the industry has long been dominated by them. Dr Imogen Shaw, a London-based general practitioner who specializes in reproductive health with particular expertise in the menopause, welcomed Guillebaud's comments and agreed that period pain has not been hugely investigated. Ignoring or dismissing reproductive health, or pain relating to it, seems to be common practice across the field of medicine. Writer Leslie Jamison also examined the ways that different forms of suffering are minimized, mocked and coaxed into silence in her essay 'Grand Unified Theory of Female Pain'. In this essay she refers to the study 'The Girl Who Cried Pain', which identified ways gender bias typically plays out in clinical pain management. In 2016, *The Independent* even reported that British men wait an average of 49 minutes before being treated for abdominal pain, whereas women will wait up to 65 minutes for the same symptoms.

I wanted to explore exactly why this is, so I spoke to Heather C. Guidone, Surgical Program Director at the Center for Endometriosis Care in Atlanta, Georgia. She agreed that stigma is definitely one of the main contributors, saying, 'Persistent shame, negative attitudes and continued reinforcement of misconceptions associated with periods continue to saturate media and society. There remains a lack of health literacy about what, when or if something is "wrong" and when to seek help. This can all potentially lead to poor practices and health outcomes.'

Guidone suffers from endometriosis herself, and believes that the doctors' mentality that running repeated failed interventions is okay still exists today. 'We should not be seeing delayed diagnoses followed by inadequate care like many of us experienced decades ago,' she explained, adding, 'We should be seeing timely referrals to expert care. In general, part of it goes back to the lack of understanding of the systemic impact of [these conditions] and how it can negatively pervade and disrupt every single aspect of an affected individual's life.'

Although Guidone and her team focus mainly on endometriosis, we spoke about a range of period-related conditions. I asked her what she thinks needs to change across the board when it comes to reproductive health. First and foremost, she said more robust research efforts that are not industry-sponsored or led by those who have never experienced a period are a must. The focus of pro-industry results means the individual isn't necessarily getting the help they need. She also stated that we are in dire need of more general awareness and education.

Think about how frequently menstrual pain (such as abdominal pain or 'cramps') is downplayed. Much like anything related to periods, cramps are still often disregarded or made fun of. Part of the problem is that pain is so normalized. (Didn't you know that cramps are supposed to be bad? It's just something we have to deal with, obviously!) People often have to go to great lengths to get their symptoms taken seriously and sometimes end up waiting years for an accurate diagnosis. For example, endometriosis-uk.org reports that there is an average of 7.5 years between people first seeing a doctor about their symptoms and receiving a firm diagnosis. They also state that 10 per cent of women of reproductive age worldwide suffer from endometriosis — that's 176 million globally. Endometriosis is the second most common gynaecological condition in the UK.

According to the United States' National Institute of Child Health and Human Development, the true number of endometriosis cases may be higher than reported, as not everyone with the condition has symptoms. If 176 million cisgender women worldwide suffer with endometriosis, then how many are suffering if we take into consideration those with other conditions (which we'll expand on later), those who have no symptoms, or anyone experiencing either of these things who isn't cisgender? That's a hell of a lot of people who might not be getting the help they need!

In addition to all this, a terrifying number of people I spoke to had experiences with doctors who had told them that the only way to manage their varying conditions was either pregnancy or a hysterectomy. Both are permanent decisions not to be taken lightly, and what happens when they're not viable options for you? We need to see a push for more answers instead of healthcare providers simply regurgitating the same outdated information. Guidone told me that there needs to be more of a focus on modern concepts, and I couldn't agree more. All this does is put people off and stops them from seeking help, because they're repeatedly hearing the same things or being turned away. This 'period pain vs heart attack' research is repeatedly reported on, with no real action following it. Perhaps if the effects of period pain were investigated further, with slightly more of a gender balance within research and medicine, this issue would finally get the necessary focus it deserves.

Of course, it's not just cramps that are as painful as some-thing that could kill us which we have to deal with during a period. My pain threshold is embarrassingly low, my boobs feel like they're made of concrete, I get uncomfortably horny, every bone in my body aches and nothing feels comfortable. Not to mention that I also feel completely drained for the first few days — and sometimes when it's over, too, as my body attempts to play catch-up. I've been men-struating for many years now and I'm still experiencing brand-new symptoms as I get older; the fun never stops! Some of the most fascinating symptoms I have experienced for the first time recent-ly include becoming completely unbalanced and falling all over the place, vulva pain (not quite like cramps; more of a dull ache but still painful), food starting to taste different and really intense nipple pain. It's also worth mentioning that a lot of PMS symptoms are not too dissimilar to early pregnancy symptoms. For example, a change in breasts, going to the toilet more often, tiredness, mood swings and changing tastes in food are all symptoms I have experienced and yet I have never had a baby or become pregnant. This could add an extra layer of stress both for people trying for a baby, and those who do not want children. People rarely consider all the different ways PMS can impact a person when mocking or dismissing those who dare to be vocal about their symptoms.

Period Poos Are Totally a Thing

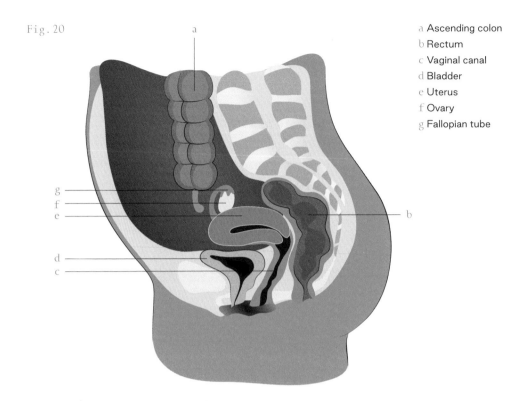

Fig. 20

a Ascending colon
b Rectum
c Vaginal canal
d Bladder
e Uterus
f Ovary
g Fallopian tube

Perhaps the most fascinating PMS symptom of all is period poos. Yep, they're a thing. A *very real* thing that doesn't get anywhere near the amount of attention it deserves! Every month, without fail, my bowels work overtime. The pain I experience, the increase in size, the consistency, it's just ridiculous. I don't know why more people aren't talking about this — I suppose most bodily functions are still quite taboo — but I'm definitely not alone. After a particularly rough period where I felt like I spent 90 per cent of my time on the toilet, I took it upon myself to do some research and find out why certain people experience this. It turns out there is actual science behind period poos! I read a ton of articles, spent countless hours trying to interpret complicated science and looked up multiple definitions. I really took one for the team, pals. Here are multiple explanations for why some of us experience an increase in bowel movements during a period:

In case you didn't know, the uterus and the colon are pretty close to one another (Fig. 20). As we've covered already, the lining of the uterus thickens over the course of the menstrual cycle. The more it thickens, the more pressure it can put on the colon. This also explains why some people feel constipated or even bloated during this time. Once things start to calm down and hormone levels start to fall, the uterus sort of begins to deflate. The pressure drops, and anything's fair game. It can become easier to poo; sometimes too easy!

→ REASON 2

Another reason involves, you guessed it, those pesky hormones again. We know progesterone helps maintain pregnancy, right? Well, as it turns out, it's also slightly constipating. It peaks right before the period, which in turn can have an effect on how our intestines process things.

If you have an influx of gas while menstruating, it's because both hormones and bacteria in the gut change during a menstrual cycle. When your body is likely experiencing fluctuating hormone levels, this can in turn make your bowels and stomach change. I'm telling you, *everything* can be blamed on hormones. *Everything.*

→ REASON 3

It could also be prostaglandins. These are natural chemicals in the body with hormone-like qualities. When released they signal the uterus to contract in order to push out the uterine lining. Now, here's where some of the reasons overlap; since the uterus and colon are so close, it's likely some head over to the bowels to wreak more havoc there. If you've ever experienced bowel cramping or feeling like you need to poo but can't, this could be why.

→ REASON 4

Stress and changes in diet could also be a factor. With things becoming tougher and cravings becoming more intense, it's only natural to be using the toilet more often. As past periods have come and gone, I've noticed which foods react well with my body and which do not. Do I stop eating them? No, I'll never learn.

My cravings during a period are some of the most intense things I've ever experienced. Sometimes I feel like I cannot function without a big bag of salty pretzels or a giant chocolate bar. There are a few possible reasons why people feel more hungry or crave comfort foods such as sweets and carbs before or during a period. One theory is that it's related to the way oestrogen and progesterone go up and then drop dramatically just before a period; another is the change in the body's response to insulin during the luteal phase. And, of course, there's also the fact that carbohydrates make us feel better when we're feeling stressed. In fact, carbs are known to promote serotonin release. Cortisol (the stress hormone) tends to spike right before a period and at the same time serotonin can dip, so it's been scientifically proven that certain foods can boost your mood. There are also certain foods that might help with PMS symptoms and some that won't, which we'll get to later (see pages 170–72). (But don't worry, you won't find any diet talk here.)

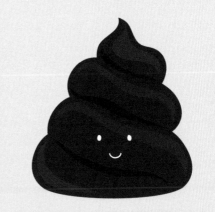

Is There Anything Good About PMS?

You may have reached a point where you're wondering, is it all bad? Do good premenstrual symptoms exist? I think some can be positive. Hear me out! Feeling everything 500 times harder than you would normally does bring certain opportunities. Having my emotions run wild has allowed me to identify what things truly upset me and ways I can handle my feelings. Each month, I get a mental reset of sorts: energy, creativity and happiness levels start to rise after my period ends and I feel almost instantly renewed. Don't get me wrong — I definitely feel relieved once my period ends (and it's totally okay to feel like you can't wait for it to be over!) — but after years of not having them I've decided that having a somewhat regular menstrual cycle is good for me mentally. They can be tough to get through, but a period essentially allows me to check in and take better care of my mental health.

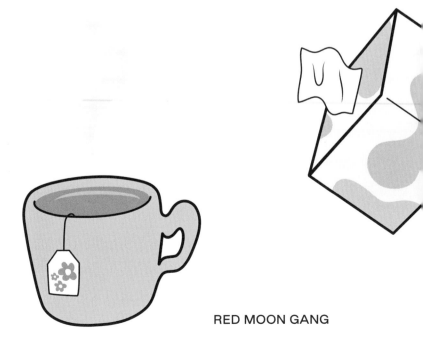

RED MOON GANG

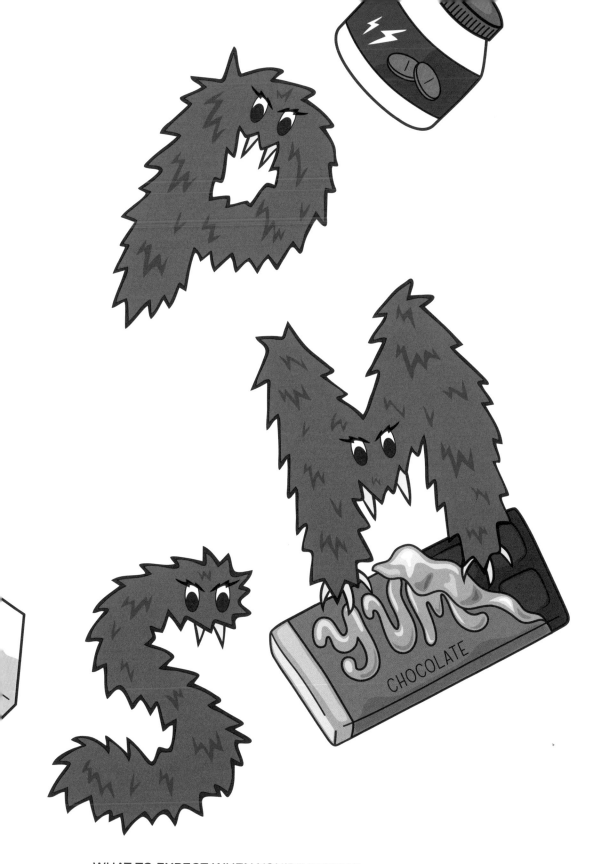

PMS, PMDD, PME — and How to Ask for Help

If you *really* struggle with your PMS symptoms there's a chance it could be something more serious, like premenstrual dysphoric disorder (PMDD). In addition to PMS, PMDD can cause extreme tension and irritability, very low self-esteem, decreased interest in normal activities, anger, anxiety and feelings of hopelessness. Depression is a common symptom and many report thoughts of suicide. Commonly defined as an endocrine disorder (meaning it's hormone-related), what makes PMDD more severe than PMS are the major mood shifts making everyday life hard to maintain. When conducting research I spoke to many who mentioned doctors failing to listen to valid concerns about the disorder. British mental health charity Mind reports that PMDD is now listed as a mental health problem in the DSM-5 (a manual doctors use to categorize and diagnose mental health issues). Hopefully this is a sign that recognition is improving, albeit slowly. It's important to remember that the intensity of any symptom can vary from body to body.

An even more rarely discussed condition is premenstrual exacerbation (PME). PMDD and PME can be difficult to distinguish from one another. PME refers to premenstrual symptoms worsening symptoms of another disorder, such as a major depressive disorder or an anxiety disorder such as post-traumatic stress disorder (PTSD), for example. It has been reported that half the people who seek treatment for PMS or PMDD actually have PME of another psychotic disorder like depression instead. More awareness and correct diagnosis that will lead to effective treatment is needed for all.

So, how can you manage these conditions? Making note of physical symptoms is just as important as the emotional effects. If you feel your pain getting worse, or your menstrual cramps are lasting longer than your period, go and see a doctor. Other signs to look out for are a change in cervical fluid; additional symptoms developing, such as a fever; symptoms in general becoming more frequent and severe; or if you feel that something is not quite right. If your period is affecting your ability to live normally, talk to your doctor immediately.

Here are some things to look out for and tips from people who have fought long and hard with doctors to have their symptoms taken seriously:

→ Gather information before you go to a doctor if you can, and try to gain a clear understanding of how your body functions. Track your periods and note all your symptoms.
→ Try to distinguish between normal and abnormal pain. Make a note of pain that is worse than your typical period pain and try implementing a pain scale.
→ When tracking on paper, colour-code each day based on heaviness of flow if you bleed a lot.
→ Note how often you have to change your period product of choice.
→ Research different conditions and see if anything stands out.
→ Seek a specialist if you aren't getting the answers you need.
→ Blood clots bigger than a large coin should be looked at.
→ If you're 30+, ask to be checked for fibroids.
→ Leaving things untreated can cause further problems; always go to the doctor the moment you think something is wrong.
→ Remember that hormonal contraception isn't the only solution, and push for other forms of treatment if this is something you wish to avoid.
→ Talk to friends and peers for comparison.

These issues are frequently dismissed, not taken seriously enough or go undiagnosed. You know when something isn't right; always push for a second opinion if you need to. If you're not at ease or don't feel happy with the outcome, you can always get a third opinion, or a fourth, and so on. It shouldn't be this way but hopefully, the more we push, the quicker things will change. Ultimately, listen to what your body tells you.

Seek a specialist, if you aren't getting the answers you're looking for

Track your periods and note all your symptoms

Talk to friends and peers for comparison

Research different conditions

Gather information before you go to a doctor

A List of Things I've Cried About While PMSing

There was no more chocolate in the house.

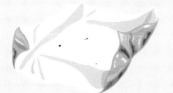

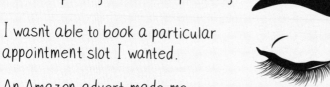

I threw up in my mouth unexpectedly.

I wasn't able to book a particular appointment slot I wanted.

An Amazon advert made me super emotional.

My cat wouldn't sit on me.

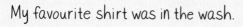

My favourite shirt was in the wash.

I needed to do a poo, but couldn't make it happen.

My partner didn't hear me.

I was really craving a certain meal, but had no energy to make it.

I burned my mouth trying to drink hot chocolate.

I couldn't find something I was looking for and it turned out it was quite literally in front of me.

Wonky eyeliner.

I sneezed and farted at the same time, and it all got a little too much.

I was completely overwhelmed by the pure density of menstrual blood exiting my body on day two.

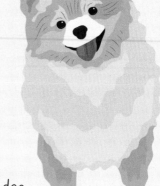

I saw a cute dog.

PERIOD CONDITIONS

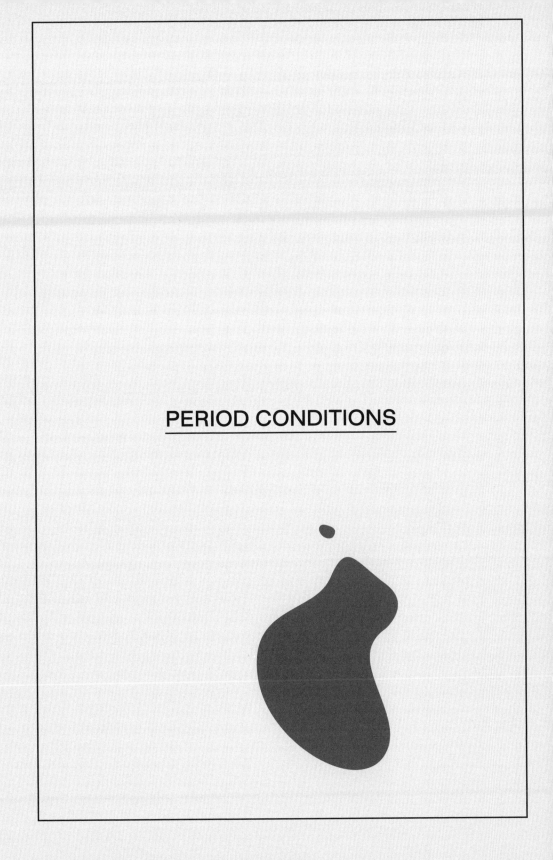

ENDOMETRIOSIS

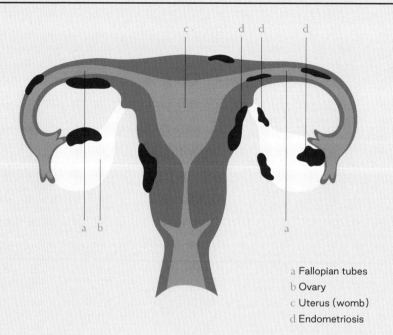

Fig. 21

a Fallopian tubes
b Ovary
c Uterus (womb)
d Endometriosis

WHAT IS IT?

A condition where tissue similar to the endometrial tissue that lines the uterus grows in other places such as the ovaries, the Fallopian tubes, around the bladder and bowel and so on. It thickens over the course of the menstrual cycle, making it incredibly painful. Many report it taking years to get a concrete diagnosis.

COMMON SYMPTOMS

- Period pain that isn't relieved with painkillers
- Heavy periods and soaking through products
- Pelvic pain
- Pain with sex, urination or bowel movements

WHAT DO DOCTORS RECOMMEND TO MANAGE IT?

- Anti–inflammatory painkillers
- Hormone medicines and contraceptives
- Surgery to get rid of patches of endometrium, or operations to remove part or all of the organs affected

WHAT DOES A 'TYPICAL' PERIOD LOOK LIKE
FOR SOMEBODY WITH ENDOMETRIOSIS?

'I'm on a pill now that regulates my periods, but I still suffer with pain. A typical period for me can last 2 to 10 days, and it's heavy from start to finish. The pain is simply unbearable and I'm usually bed-bound for the first two days. Sometimes the blood used to be really dark or even black, but I have since learned that this was due to an infection caused by the endometriosis. I have to wear large sanitary pads intended for night time all the time.'
– H, 29.

'I've had a lot of different treatments. I was on the pill at 15, which meant having a more regular cycle. I was able to go to school, but still experienced a great amount of pain. At 23, I decided to come off the pill as it had stopped me from living a "normal" teenage life. I also started to experience a lot of ovulation pain mid-cycle; I ended up in hospital one time because of it. My sex drive made an appearance when I reached 24. From the age of 24 to 35, I managed my periods with mefenamic acid as well as tranexamic acid. From 30 onwards, incidents of flooding increased. By 35, the bleeding had reached a whole new excessive level. I had unbearable pain throughout my entire menstrual cycle and soiled myself twice at work. I had an endometrial ablation via electrocoagulation at 35. They insert very thin tools through your vagina to reach your uterus; in my case they used an electrical mesh. This expands, and then the energy and heat sent by radio waves damage the lining, which is then removed with suction. I bled lightly for about six weeks after, then my periods stopped completely for three years. I'm 40 now and my periods are back, but they're a lot lighter. I have a more regular cycle of 26 days, and my period only lasts for five days or so. Now I only need to wear a regular pad! I still have some pain, but nothing like what I used to have.'
– B, 40.

POLYCYSTIC OVARY SYNDROME (PCOS)

Fig. 22

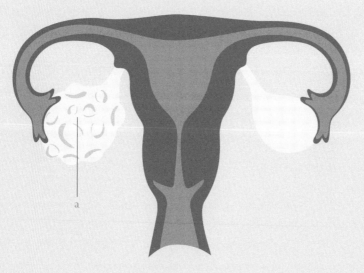

a Polycystic ovary

WHAT IS IT?

A condition that affects hormone levels and how the ovaries and ovulation work. Some people with PCOS produce higher-than-normal amounts of androgens such as testosterone, which in turn disrupts the menstrual cycle. In many cases, small cysts grow on the ovaries. The eggs never mature enough to trigger ovulation, making it harder to conceive.

COMMON SYMPTOMS

- Irregular periods
- Heavy bleeding as the uterine lining builds up for a longer amount of time
- Hair growth, particularly on the face, chest, belly or back
- Acne
- Weight gain
- Headaches
- Darkening of the skin
- Hair thinning

WHAT DO DOCTORS RECOMMEND TO MANAGE IT?

- Lifestyle changes such as diet or weight loss
- Contraceptive pills and other medicines that help regulate the menstrual cycle and treat PCOS symptoms like hair growth and acne
- Metformin, a drug used to treat type 2 diabetes that also helps manage PCOS by improving insulin levels
- Fertility drugs to help those with PCOS get pregnant
- Hair removal medicines
- Surgery to help restore regular ovulation and improve fertility

WHAT DOES A 'TYPICAL' PERIOD LOOK LIKE FOR SOMEBODY WITH PCOS?

'My period comes at any time; the gap can be anything from three to six weeks. Before I had cysts removed, my periods were really painful. I've collapsed on the Tube before, unable to walk and close to vomiting from pain. It was common for me to lie on the sofa crying on the first day. They were also incredibly heavy. I would put a pad on and I'd be ready to change within the hour.' – J, 28.

'The biggest gap between periods I've experienced was about 11 weeks, which was really unusual for me. When my periods do come, they last about three days. I get horrific mood swings about 7 to 10 days before the period. I'll go from being calm and collected to enraged in seconds. I get really bad pain in my lower back and abdomen for the first day. Occasionally, I won't be able to get out of bed. However, this only ever happens on the first day. I'll feel uncomfortable, restless and twitchy throughout.' – B, 33.

'As I do not consistently ovulate, PMS can seem to last for weeks. When I do ovulate I can feel a twinge in my ovaries at the point of ovulation and the period that follows can be very heavy. I was very in touch with my cycle prior to developing PCOS, and find that not knowing when my period is coming is quite disorienting. My cycles can vary in length from 28 to 120 days. My PMS has started to worsen over time; I can get so bloated I vomit and find that I grow a lot more facial hair and get a lot more spots in the run-up to my period. I am unable to go on the pill to regulate my periods as it interacts with other medical conditions I have. I'm learning to live with the irregularity and unpredictability of my periods, but sometimes I would rather they were regular and predictable again.' – S, 34.

PREMENSTRUAL DYSPHORIC DISORDER (PMDD)

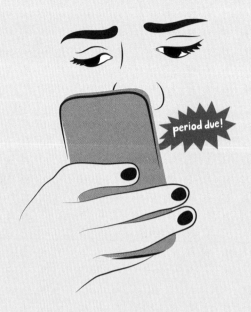

WHAT IS IT?

A severe form of PMS with symptoms that are much worse and have a serious impact on your life. PMDD can make it difficult to work and socialize. In many cases it can also lead to suicidal thoughts.

COMMON SYMPTOMS

- Severe depression symptoms; feelings of hopelessness or self-deprecating thoughts
- Irritability and tension before menstruation builds up for a longer amount of time
- Difficulty concentrating, feeling overwhelmed, lack of energy and less interest in activities you normally enjoy
- Other overwhelming physical symptoms such as breast tenderness or swelling, headaches, etc.
- Suicidal feelings

WHAT DO DOCTORS RECOMMEND TO MANAGE IT?

- Antidepressants (SSRIs)
- Hormonal contraception to help regulate cycles
- Psychotherapy such as cognitive behavioural therapy (CBT)

WHAT DOES A 'TYPICAL' PERIOD LOOK LIKE FOR SOMEBODY WITH PMDD?

'A typical cycle off the pill involves suicidal ideation and potential self-harming in the run-up to my period. When it does arrive, it's followed by excruciating pain for eight days while feeling incredibly depressed and craving random foods. On the pill, my period is a lot better. I still feel depressed during the time leading up to it, but it's not so severe or dangerous. My periods are still very painful, but I can usually manage a few active days. They now only last for seven days, as opposed to eight or more.' — B, 26.

'As soon as ovulation occurs my energy and mood start to drop, and I get more reclusive. The PMDD symptoms usually show around two to three days before my period, but can sometimes be as early as 5 to 10 days. I am irritated more easily and I'm also extremely fatigued. About two days before, I have issues with conflict. I am prone to crying and experience feelings of hopelessness as well as suicidal thoughts. If I am already dealing with things that are troubling me, this can be a dangerous time.' — K, 27.

'At first, my GP tried to establish if there were any "logical" reasons for the way I was feeling. There was nothing to report and she asked me to wait another month to see if the same pattern occurred, which it did. She then tried to convince me that this is something everyone with a period experiences. I listened to my intuition and kept return-ing to see her until she believed it was more than regular PMS and the stress of parenting. I had multiple tests and they all came back fine. It was at this time I just completely broke down; I simply would not accept that this was all in my head. I had already self-diagnosed by staying up countless nights and Googling my symptoms in the hope of getting to the bottom of this. PMDD was the condition that resonated the strongest with me. My GP started to take me more seriously the moment I broke down in her office; she grabbed a book and checked the symptoms of PMDD. Why did it take a breakdown for my GP to seriously look into my symptoms?' — L, 28.

MENORRHAGIA

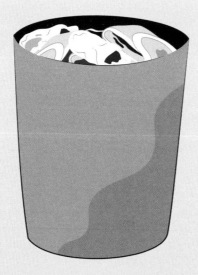

WHAT IS IT?

The medical term for periods that come with abnormally heavy or prolonged bleeding.

COMMON SYMPTOMS

- Flow lasting longer than seven days
- Having to change your product of choice very frequently (every one to two hours, for example)
- Blood clots that are the size of a large coin
- Possible anaemia due to the volume of blood loss
- Inability to perform everyday activities because of the bleeding

IS DIAGNOSIS EASIER?

It seems as though diagnosis is a bit more straightforward in this case. Most of the people I spoke with about it were able to be diagnosed just by having their blood looked at. One person in particular said their GP noticed they had low iron levels and they were diagnosed with anaemia and menorrhagia there and then!

WHAT DOES A 'TYPICAL' PERIOD LOOK LIKE FOR SOMEBODY WITH MENORRHAGIA?

'Every month, it feels like life is trying to leave my body through my uterus. I have constant stabbing pain for five days a month. No one believed me when I said my pain was agonizing until I pleaded and described it as labour pain.' — S, 33.

'Before my hysterectomy, my periods were really irregular. I'd have one every two weeks for a couple of months, then they would disap–pear for about three months. The pain from cramps was like no pain I had ever experienced before. The cramps would appear so suddenly and they would leave me doubled over and screaming on the floor. My periods would be so heavy, there would be lots of blood clots and I would soak through pads. It made my life impossible.' — R, 30.

ADENOMYOSIS

Fig. 23

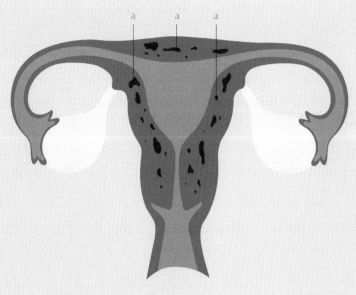

a Adenomyosis

WHAT IS IT?

A condition where the endometrium breaks through the uterus's muscle wall (the myo-metrium) and the uterus becomes inflamed in response. It can sometimes be hard to distinguish between adenomyosis and endometriosis by symptoms alone. Before technology advanced, the only sure way to diagnose adenomyosis was to perform a hysterectomy and examine the uterus once it had been removed!

COMMON SYMPTOMS

- Heavy, prolonged bleeding
- Severe menstrual cramps
- Abdominal pressure and bloating

WHAT DO DOCTORS RECOMMEND TO MANAGE IT?

- Taking NSAIDs one to two days before the beginning of a period and continuing through the first few days
- Hormonal therapies such as the IUD (intrauterine device, also known as a coil) and the contraceptive injection
- Uterine artery embolization, a minimally invasive procedure that guides particles through a tiny tube into the patient's femoral artery; with the blood supply cut off, the adenomyosis can shrink
- Endometrial ablation, a procedure that destroys the lining of the uterus and can be effective when adenomyosis hasn't penetrated deeply into the muscle wall

WHAT DOES A 'TYPICAL' PERIOD LOOK LIKE
FOR SOMEBODY WITH ADENOMYOSIS?

'We went through a trial and error process. The contraceptive injec-tion was recommended first, as this normally stops periods. I tried it for nine months and I absolutely hated everything about it; I had terrible mood swings, zero sex drive and sex itself took a lot of work. As I was discharged once I'd received a diagnosis, I went back to a family planning clinic. They put me on the progesterone–only pill instead, which I now take continuously back to back without any breaks. It has changed my life; I have no pain and I can live my life again without dreading and planning for my period.' — G, 26.

'It feels like I am having contractions every month without the baby afterwards. Stabbing pains I can only describe as sharp shocks. I can't move, I can't do anything, I just feel like my world is shutting down. The blood is so heavy, every month is a struggle and it has gotten progressively worse over the years. I have lost so much blood; I change my clothes on average three times a day and I've had to have a blood transfusion. I'm not old enough to be considered for a hysterectomy and I am more than ready.' — S, 41.

DYSMENORRHEA

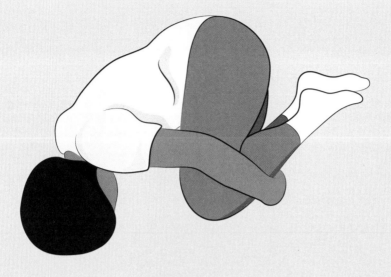

WHAT IS IT?

The medical term given to pain with menstruation. There are two types. Primary dysmenorrhea is typical menstrual cramps that are recurrent and not due to other conditions. Secondary dysmenorrhea is pain that is caused by another condition in the reproductive organs (such as endo-metriosis or adenomyosis). Secondary dysmenorrhea usually begins earlier in the menstrual cycle and lasts longer than typ-ical menstrual cramps.

COMMON SYMPTOMS

- Aching pain in the abdomen (may be severe at times)
- Feeling of pressure in the abdomen
- Pain in the hips, lower back and inner thighs

WHAT DO DOCTORS RECOMMEND TO MANAGE IT?

- NSAIDs and hormonal contraception
- Lifestyle changes and general PMS advice, like applying heat
- Mefenamic acid

WHAT HAS LED PEOPLE TO GET THEIR PERIOD LOOKED AT?

'I got my first period when I was 12 and it was pretty uneventful. About eight months later, it was a completely different ball game. I was in agony; standard painkillers did nothing, they didn't even take the edge off. Both my mum and gran suffered with dysmenorrhea and my mum instantly recognized the symptoms. We hoped it would be a one-off and battled through. About four months after that, I got my third period and it was unbearable. The pain was like nothing I've ever experienced, and I've since given birth!' – S, 41.

'What led me to get my periods looked at initially was the intensity of pain as well as how irregular they were. I would bleed at least twice every month for three to four days at a time and it was more than spotting. I had been on the mini-pill for four years and hadn't had any problems with my periods. The irregularity and pain contin-ued for six months, so I went to see somebody who specializes in sexual health and contraception.' – L, 25.

'I have always had painful periods for as long as I can remember. When I was younger, I would complain about the pain and the amount of blood. I would be dismissed for a number of reasons; mostly people thought I was exaggerating. I also had no measure of what was "normal" as periods were new to me and my friends didn't share their experiences. It wasn't until I had to skip school and social outings that my mum suggested we look into it in further detail.' – H, 22.

FIBROIDS

Fig. 24

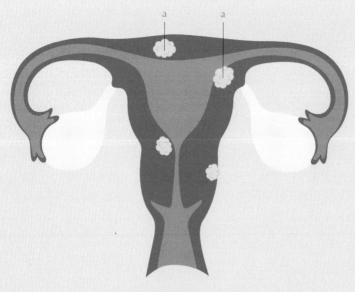

a Fibroids

WHAT IS IT?

Fibroids are non-cancerous growths that develop in or around the uterus. They can vary in size and do not always come with symptoms.

COMMON SYMPTOMS

- Heavy or painful periods
- Abdominal pain
- Lower back pain
- Frequent need to urinate
- Pain or discomfort during sex
- Constipation

WHAT DO DOCTORS RECOMMEND TO MANAGE THEM?

- IUD to stop the lining of the uterus growing quickly
- Tranexamic acid to stop the small blood vessels in the uterine lining bleeding, reducing blood loss
- NSAIDs that can reduce the body's production of prostaglandin
- The contraceptive pill; oral and injected progestogen
- Medication to shrink fibroids
- Surgery to remove fibroids if symptoms are particularly severe and medication has been ineffective

STORIES THAT PROVE DOCTORS NEED TO DO BETTER BY THEIR PATIENTS

'My periods started getting more painful a few years back. I couldn't concentrate at work and would often spend days at home in pain. When painkillers were not working, my doctor suggested I get the implant. I had to have it taken out after a month, though, as my periods got progressively worse. I would bleed for weeks on end and would get through roughly six to seven packs of pads a day. I was eventually taken into hospital for a blood transfusion; I was prescribed codeine, mefenamic and tranexamic acid. They stopped the bleeding, but I was still in constant pain every day. I could just about make it to work, but I could barely sit down. This went on for over a year until the doctors eventually agreed to operate and find out what was wrong. I had been in hospital for two blood transfusions previously, which means an endless number of appointments and scans. They found a small fibroid, but everything else came back clear. Once they came to operate they found that the fibroid had grown so large that it had caused a prolapsed uterus. This explains why I had trouble sitting down.' – N, 36.

'I was diagnosed with endometriosis five years ago and fibroids just a year ago. I felt familiar endo symptoms returning, but also found I had a very firm lump in my abdomen. It made sitting up, lying on my front or standing for too long extremely painful. My fibroid is around the size of a four-month-old foetus. I had four appointments with six different doctors before I was diagnosed; it took well over a year. Although the doctors were always professional, they were not the most sympathetic. I've had issues with endometriosis since I was 12 and recurring issues even since surgery. I'm tired. I'm tired of it all and consistently worried about what is going to come next. Doctors don't seem to care or acknowledge my history. Every treatment I experience is considered with fertility in mind, despite me saying that my focus is being healthy and not fertile. The prospect of a fictional child is more of a priority to doctors than my rapidly declining health.' – S, 27.

'During my twenties, my periods got so bad I couldn't go anywhere or do anything. I was in incredible pain and, after my laparoscopy, the doctor told me I had endometriosis. They told me the best thing for it was to get pregnant. I wish I could tell you I was joking. It was very frustrating.' — K, 41.

'I've had PCOS, endometriosis, adenomyosis and fibroids. Had increasingly excruciating periods from age 11 up until I finally got a hysterectomy at age 30. I researched and already suspected I had endo by my late teens — and was already more than willing to get a hysterectomy by that point, as I already knew I never wanted to have a child. I saw a lot of different GPs and gynaecologists over the years. The most outrageous was the male gynae who told me that God intended for women to be in pain, and yelled at me for complaining.' — N, 39.

'When I was a medical student, I went to my GP after I'd not had a period for 3 months... Cue roughly 6 months of "are you sure you're not pregnant?" After 18 months, the male GP's response was "Why do you care? I though women hated periods?" Well. Yes. But it's abnormal, and therefore scary.' — F, 34.

'I've had periods for almost 10 years. In that time they have always been extremely heavy, painful and irregular. I've consistently been told the cause of this won't be investigated, as my diet/lifestyle/contraception choice is probably the cause, aka it's my own fault.' — F, 23.

PERIOD

PRO-
DUCTS

Decisions, Decisions

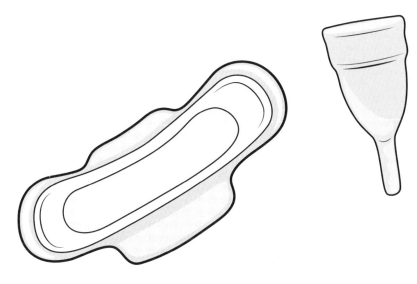

Growing up, I struggled immensely with period products. Although my uterus has been wild and unruly since the day it sprang into action, one thing I could always count on was a heavy flow. And when I first started menstruating, the only two viable options were tampons that robbed me of any moisture and pads that felt like itchy nappies. I experimented with different brands, styles, sizes, absorbencies — but it didn't matter what I tried, everything irritated me in its own unique way. My knowledge of alternatives was non-existent and, for a very long time, I thought this was just how periods were meant to be: long, pointless, uncomfortable and miserable.

Fortunately a lot has changed since then, and I have since discovered a wealth of innovative products and options. Now, I can't help but wonder how much easier navigating my periods would have been if I had found out about these products sooner. If you're currently struggling with products, wanting to reduce plastic waste or even just curious, here's a rundown on all the period products I've tried, myth- and misinformation-free!

PAD	DIFFERENT STYLES

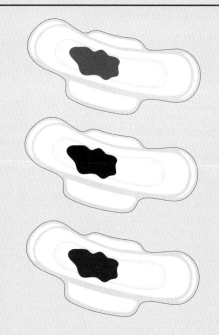

HOW DO YOU USE IT?

- Externally. Sits between vulva and underpants and collects blood.

HOW OFTEN DO YOU CHANGE IT?

- Every three to four hours, or when it's soaked with blood
- If you're changing it every hour, see a doctor

HOW DO YOU DISPOSE OF IT?

- Fold it over, wrap it up in the packaging it comes in and pop it in the designated bins commonly found next to a toilet in public bathrooms.
- Put it in one of those small disposable waste bags or simply wrap it in toilet paper and put it in your regular bin. Never flush!

DIFFERENT STYLES

- Panty liner: These are marketed for daily cervical fluid, light menstrual flow and spotting, as well as slight urinary incontinence. Can be worn towards the end of a period on days when you're not sure if it's over or not.
- Ultra-thin: This is a thin pad mainly used by people who worry about bulk and their pads being visible. They can be just as absorbent as regular or super pads.
- Regular: Your standard run-of-the-mill pad; these are a good middle ground in terms of absorbency.
- Super/maxi: These are useful for people with heavy flows, as they are normally on the higher end of the absorbency scale.
- Overnight: These pads are longer and intended for overnight use, as they allow more protection while lying down. (There has been more than one occasion when I've had to use this type of pad during the day, and I don't think I'm alone here.)
- Maternity: Slightly longer than super/maxi pads, these absorb bleeding that occurs after childbirth. They can also absorb urine.
- Other: Some pads come with 'wings' that enable you to keep them in place around your underwear. 'Wingless' pads exist too. Some retailers also sell additional ranges with features that supposedly absorb more or vary in size, such as 'ultra-long' pads.

PROS	CONS
• Available in a range of styles covering every type of need from panty liners and regular everyday pads to overnight, maxi and even urinary incontinence pads • Found in a lot of shops including pound shops and supermarkets • Different designs available, like 'wingless' (those who wear them are the bravest of all!) • Non-penetrative; no insertion needed • Safe for overnight use • Organic and fragrance-free options available	• Still largely unattainable for many; overpriced and not enough in one pack to last a cycle • Companies are not obliged to disclose harmful ingredients that go into their products • Plastic, porous material often made from wood or polyester fibre and paper pulp are some of the most commonly found ingredients • Adhesive can sometimes give you an unexpected pubic waxing! • Often bleached to appear white and sprayed with perfumes and artificial fragrances that can upset the vagina's delicate pH balance • Generate a lot of waste that ends up in landfill or in oceans and rivers and on beaches

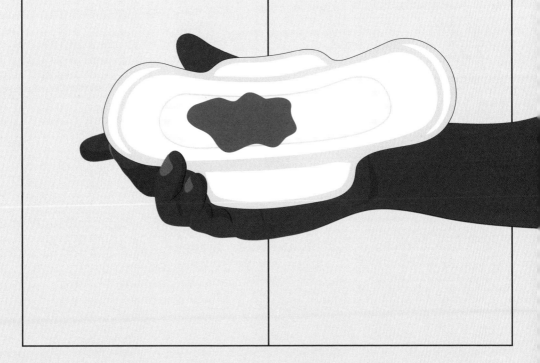

TAMPON

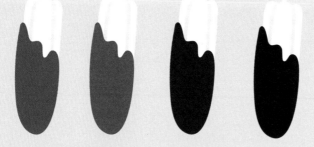

HOW DO YOU USE IT?

- Internally. Absorbs menstrual flow when inserted into the vagina.

HOW OFTEN DO YOU CHANGE IT?

- Every four hours; don't leave for longer than eight
- Use the lowest absorbency tampon needed for your flow. Using a super absorbent tampon on your lightest days can increase your risk of Toxic Shock Syndrome (TSS), a rare but dangerous condition caused by bacterial toxins
- If you're changing it every hour, see a doctor

HOW DO YOU DISPOSE OF IT?

- Never flush! Simply wrap it up and throw it in the bin along with the wrapper and applicator (if any).

DIFFERENT STYLES

- Applicator: Tampon with a string and applicator. The latter consists of two tubes to help you insert the tampon; the outer tube is like a barrel of sorts and the second is the inner tube — think of it like a plunger. There's a gap in this tube for the tampon to sit on to be pushed inside you. Once the plunger meets your vulva and the tampon is in, the two tubes become one and have served their purpose.
- Non-applicator: Tampon that is inserted into the vaginal canal with a finger (or reusable applicator).
- Other: Some retailers sell tampons with features that are supposed to help with absorbency, such as expanding lengthways. However, they're often very drying.

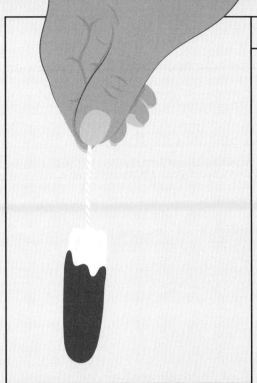

- Can be hard to know if you're wearing it correctly; that awkward waddle you do after putting in a tampon seems to be a rite of passage
- Can be hard to insert
- Once you *do* have it down, they can be very easy to forget about
- Although nowadays it is rare, people who use tampons are most at risk of getting Toxic Shock Syndrome (TSS)
- Often highly absorbent, as the vagina maintains a delicate balance of good and bad bacteria — sometimes tampons absorb the good stuff
- Often made from highly absorbent viscose rayon, which is one of many synthetic ingredients commonly associated with the likelihood of TSS; also many are heavily fragranced and, again, brands don't have to list what chemicals they're using
- Chlorine is often used in the bleaching process and produces trace amounts of dioxins, which have been linked to hormone disruption and can affect people's immune systems. According to the Environmental Protection Agency, there is no safe level of exposure to dioxins, plus we have no idea what the long-term effects of exposure could be
- Still largely unattainable for many, with machines that stock them providing very few for an extortionate price and with period products (most notably tampons) being taxed as non-essential 'luxury' items, referred to as the 'tampon tax'
- Contribute to an enormous amount of waste that cannot be broken down and ends up in landfill or in oceans and rivers and on beaches
- Although not frequently discussed, fibre loss is something to be aware of (pro tip: put a tampon in a glass of water to test how much it comes apart)

PROS

- Available in several absorbency ratings, as well as different designs (such as with applicator or without)
- Easy to transport if you're somebody who is embarrassed about menstru-ating (although you don't need to be!)
- If you ask someone for a tampon and they don't have one, they will not rest until they find you one — it's just an unspoken law
- Found in most supermarkets and other high-street shops
- No uncomfortable wet feeling if you're unable to change right away
- Offers more freedom of movement (i.e. athletic activities) if placed correctly
- Organic and fragrance-free options available, as well as plastic-free applicators

SOFTCUP / MENSTRUAL DISC

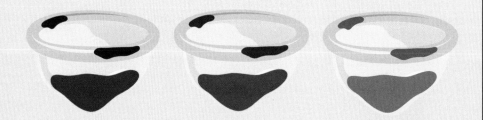

HOW DO YOU USE IT?

- Internally. Collects menstrual flow by insertion into the vagina.
- If you feel something in the vaginal canal, it is not in far enough; remove it and try again by sliding it back and tilting it slightly downwards.

HOW OFTEN DO YOU CHANGE IT?

- Every six hours depending on your flow; do not leave longer than 12 hours

HOW DO YOU DISPOSE OF IT?

- Empty menstrual fluid into a toilet or sink.
- Put it into the wrapper or wrap in toilet paper, and throw it in the bin.

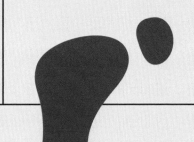

RED MOON GANG

PROS	CONS
• Sits closer to the cervix to collect blood, which means less risk of leaking • Great introduction to alternative products and offers a first taste of menstrual cups • Different shape to reusable menstrual cups that could be easier for some • Can be worn for up to 12 hours • Insertion can potentially be easier than for reusable menstrual cups as all you need to do is squeeze the rim together, making it a similar shape to a tampon, as opposed to trying different folding methods • There is also a reusable version available, Intimina's Ziggy Cup	• Will need to be changed more frequently if you have a heavy flow • Not many brands currently available on the market, and it can be difficult to obtain the amount you're after without committing to a subscription service • Can be hard to figure out how many you need per cycle • Different shape to reusable menstrual cups that could be hard to get used to

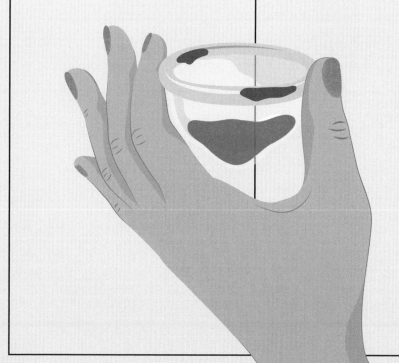

CLOTH PAD	DIFFERENT STYLES

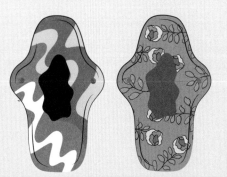

DIFFERENT STYLES

- All-in-one: This is the most common form that cloth pads take. The pad is absorbent and may have waterproofing sewn into it. Simply put it in your underpants and you're ready to go.
- Pocket: This is an empty pad-shaped shell that has an opening where separate removable items known as 'inserts' or 'boosters' are placed. This is good for people with unpredictable flows, as you can adjust the amount of absorbency and the thickness of the pad.
- Base and insert: These have a 'base' pad that comes with absorbent inserts that are placed on top. The inserts can attach in a number of ways, including snaps, buttons, Velcro or even straps. Sometimes, the base is underwear. You can change the inserts while leaving the base, so they come in handy on days when you need to change more regularly. The inserts also take up less room when travelling.
- Foldable: These pads include a section that folds out for quicker drying. They usually feature a winged pad shape sewn to a large rectangle or square that is then folded into thirds to form the absorbent part of the pad.
- Boostable: Similar to the base and insert, these pads range in absorbency but can provide additional coverage too. The only difference is that these can function as pads with or without a boost, whereas pocket pads, for example, are generally an empty shell.

HOW DO YOU USE IT?

- Externally. Sits between vulva and underpants and collects blood.

HOW OFTEN DO YOU CHANGE IT?

- As often as you would disposable pads/whenever you need to

HOW DO YOU DISPOSE OF IT?

- You don't!
- Simply wash and reuse (head to page 176 for cleaning tips).

PROS	CONS
• Typically made with materials that are 'breathable' and more comfortable as well as quick-drying and highly absorbent, such as bamboo • Always on hand: no more having to take emergency trips to the shops • Say goodbye to 'waxing' as there is no adhesive strip to catch pubic hair, and less chance of causing irritation altogether • Reusable and zero waste; cheaper than disposables in the long run • Feel softer than plastic/paper disposables • Huge range of colourful fabrics and patterns available • More choice in terms of shape, style and absorbency options • More absorbent, and some find they need to be changed less frequently • Some people also find they are likely to change their pad more often with cloth, as they don't have to worry about 'wasting' a disposable pad • Can wash them in the washing machine; many styles can be tumble-dried • Some styles have waterproofing sewn in, making them more leakproof than disposables • Some styles can resist staining and many find no issue with staining anyway • No bin full of used pads sitting in the bathroom • Many brands donate to those in need	• More expensive to purchase initially; it can take time to figure out what works for you, how many you need and to build a collection • Can feel bulkier if you're somebody who prefers 'ultra-thin' styles • Not as readily available, as they're not stocked in mainstream supermarkets • You have to buy a lot of them or do a lot of washing to make it through a period relying solely on cloth pads • Take time to wash and dry; people may feel embarrassed using them around people they live with or not have space to use them privately • Disposable pads are quicker and easier to use • Can shift around more than disposables • Many people find the concept unpleasant • You have to bring used cloth pads home with you if you change them while you're out (although wet bags are available)

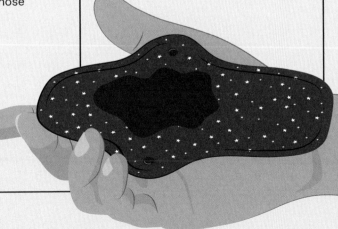

MENSTRUAL CUP

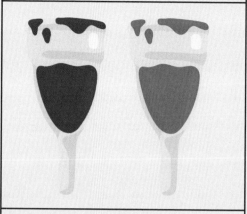

HOW DO YOU USE IT?

- Internally. Collects menstrual flow by insertion into the vagina.

HOW OFTEN DO YOU CHANGE IT?

- As often as you need to
- Try emptying it every two to four hours until you get a good sense of how full your cup gets; chances are you'll only need to change it a few times a day

HOW DO YOU DISPOSE OF IT?

- You don't!
- Sterilize and reuse (see page 176 for cleaning tips).

ANATOMY OF A MENSTRUAL CUP

- Rim: The top opening of the cup
- Suction holes: Pin-sized holes that can be found just below the rim. Although they're often referred to as suction holes, they're more like anti-suction holes. They help break the seal and prevent suction during removal. Some cups have them, some don't
- Stem: The small part that sticks out from the bottom of the cup. Like cups, stems can vary. There are slim ones, thick ones, hollow ones, solid ones and even cups that have a ring stem. Unlike a tampon string, which is visible, this sits inside you. It can also be trimmed or removed completely; some people with lower cervixes trim the stem so it's not sticking out. I wouldn't recommend altering the stem until you know you need to as, ultimately, it's there to help you extract the cup with ease
- Base: The bottom of the cup, just above the stem
- Seam/seamless: Finally, some cups have seams down the side of the cup from the mould used to make them. There are others that are seamless and smooth.

DIFFERENT FOLDS FOR INSERTION

- C Fold (also known as the U Fold): Fold your cup in half so the lips of the rim touch, then slowly bend the cup in half again lengthwise. At the point of insertion, the cup will resemble a C or a U depending on what way you hold it. (Note: although this is the method most commonly recommended by menstrual cup companies, it's actually the fold that makes the menstrual cup widest at the point of insertion. So if you're struggling to get it in, that may be why.)
- Punchdown Fold (also known as the Shell Fold): Hold your menstrual cup and use your thumb to push the rim of the cup down towards the base. Remove your thumb as you squeeze the edges together. (Note: The Punchdown Fold creates one of the smallest areas of insertion. Some can find the cup difficult to 'pop' open correctly. Try inserting the fold partway, letting it open and then pushing the remainder of the way.)

- 7 Fold (also known as the Triangle Fold): Fold your menstrual cup in half so the lips of the rim touch, then pull down on the right side to form a 7 shape. To make the triangle version, bring the right corner down towards the base of the cup. (Note: This fold 'pops' open easier than the Punchdown Fold.)
- Origami Fold: Hold your menstrual cup upright and push the front lip halfway down inside the cup (not quite as far as you would using the Punchdown Fold). Take the right corner of the cup and bring it down to the base of the left side.

Whichever fold you decide to try, hold the folded sides and insert in an upwards motion. Do it slowly and aim to keep your muscles relaxed. If you need to stop and start again, that's totally okay! Bodies are weird: some days it's easy and sometimes it's the hardest thing in the world to do. Try not to get disheartened and just keep practising. I highly recommend using a water–based lube to make insertion easier. I use a small dollop and rub it around the rim. If you have a high cervix, you can use the stem to push the cup further up once the base is in.

PROS

- Just one initial cost as opposed to buying products every month
- Designed for long–term use, with some cups lasting up to 10 years
- Less landfill waste; some cups are even biodegradable
- Made with material that doesn't upset the vagina and its delicate pH balance
- More time between changes; can be worn for up to 12 hours
- Huge range of designs for different cervix heights and menstrual needs
- Can help people view menstruation in a different light
- Have been known to help with cramps, make flow more manageable and eliminate blood clots
- In 2019, medical journal *The Lancet* found that menstrual cups are as safe and effective as other options. This included an analysis of 43 studies and 3,319 participants, making this the largest and most comprehensive review of menstrual cups to date!

CONS

- Expensive; costs can add up if you have to try multiple cups
- Insertion and removal can be tricky and take practice
- Can take a while to get used to it or to know if it's right for you; many brands recommend sticking with it for up to three cycles
- Users have more contact with blood
- Can be messy, especially if you are inexperienced
- Require maintenance after each cycle that some people may not be able to do, such as sterilizing
- There have been stories of people dislodging their IUD while trying to remove their cup (the trick is to ask your GP to clip the IUD strings short so they don't get in the way, and to be extra careful when releasing the suction before pulling your cup to take it out)

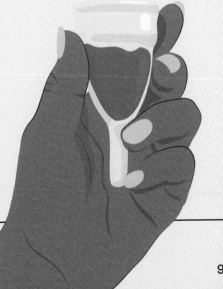

PERIOD UNDERWEAR

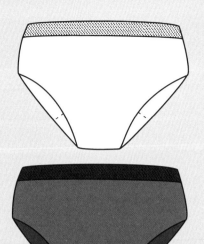

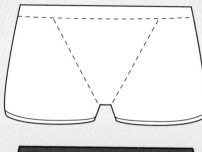

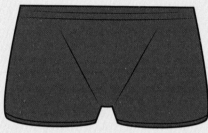

HOW DO YOU USE IT?

- Wear it. Absorbs menstrual fluid.

HOW OFTEN DO YOU CHANGE IT?

- However often you need to
- Wear once, wash and reuse

HOW DO YOU DISPOSE OF IT?

- You don't! (Again, you can find cleaning tips on page 176).

RED MOON GANG

PROS	CONS
• Offer leak-proof protection • More comfortable than other products • Many fashion-friendly styles available • Can save money in the long run • Some brands have a pouch at the front so you can hold a heating pad or pain management device to ease cramps • Often anti-microbial, meaning they kill bacteria • You don't have to worry about products moving around • Most brands are very absorbent and you don't have to worry about changing throughout the day (unless your flow is particularly heavy) • Lots of styles out there; many brands have products that can be worn during athletic activities without the worry of leaking (such as ModiBodi's activewear) • Many brands offer discounts regularly, particularly if you build a cycle set	• Often very expensive; it can be hard to afford to buy a whole cycle set in one go • Availability differs from country to country and shipping raises costs • You have to buy a lot of them or do a lot of washing to make it through a period relying solely on period underwear • Some brands are not as absorbent as others and work better as a backup to an internal method like a tampon or menstrual cup • Brands that are less absorbent can offer a feeling of 'wetness' • Plus-size people are often forgotten in terms of size; ModiBodi (26) and Flux (28/30) offer the largest • Should be rinsed immediately after use (can be left to dry out before washing, though) • Can lose their shape in the wash if a delicates bag isn't used

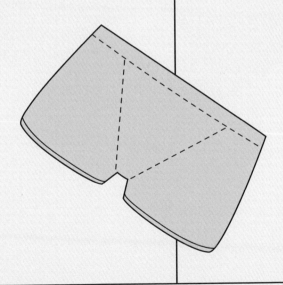

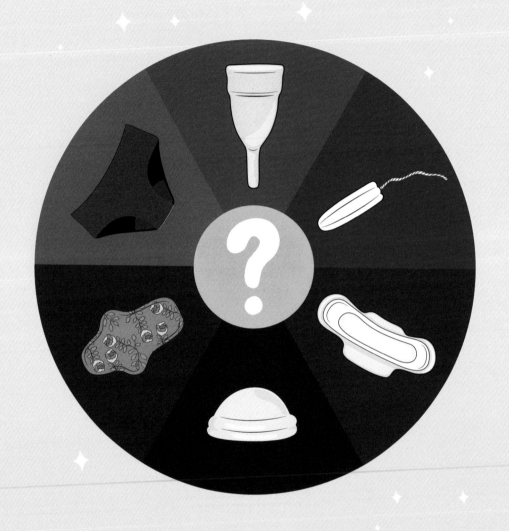

PERIODS

SEX

AND

One of Life's Greatest Pleasures

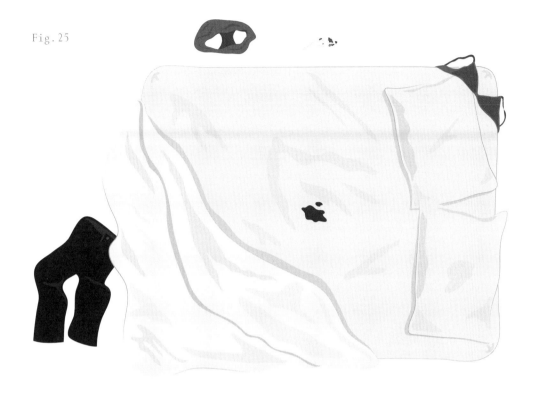

Fig. 25

I'm going to go out on a limb here and say that — for people of an appropriate age — period sex is one of the greatest pleasures life has to offer. Although you're not *supposed* to feel horniest when you're least fertile, as it's not in your body's best interest to get it on during this time, sexual urges don't just magically disappear because somebody is on their period. Shock horror! And I'll let you in on a little secret, too: more people than you realize are participating in this taboo–breaking act; they're just not talking about it. Unless you're especially squeamish, there's no need to avoid sexual activity during a period. Although it can be a bit messy (Fig. 25), it's perfectly safe. If this is a topic that makes you uncomfortable or you're not yet sex-ually active, you may want to skip ahead, which reminds me — loved ones, if you don't want to read about me in an explicit context, look away now!

Feeling empowered plays a big part in why I enjoy period sex so much. Personally, me and period sex go way back. I spent years failing to recognize that an impossible-to-scratch itch I would experience near the beginning of each period was in fact arousal. Once I did, I spent even more time wrestling with the fact that I am probably my horniest in all my menstruating glory. I unearthed these desires during my awkward teen phase when my peers and the people I slept with were all just as angsty, shame-riddled and clueless as I was. It was a very confusing time. When I finally reached the acceptance stage, there was nobody around to have sex with. It's been a long, tedious and frankly exhausting journey, which is why period sex is now something I cherish (Fig. 26). It's a time when I can completely let go, relax and enjoy some good old-fashioned, unadulterated pleasure.

Fig. 26

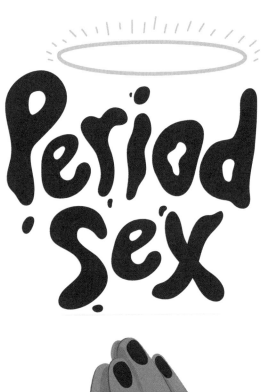

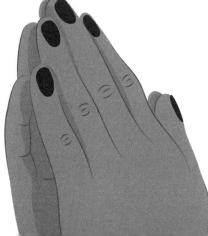

Outdated Ideals Deprive People of Pleasure

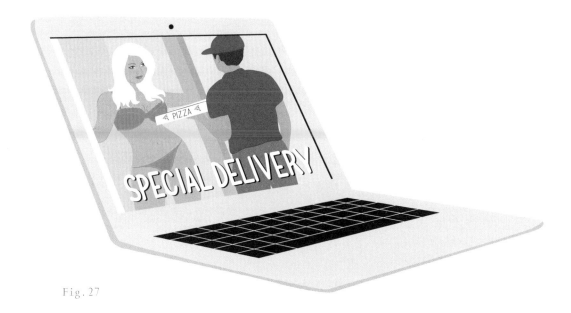

Fig. 27

As we've established already, periods have been unfairly framed as disgusting and unnatural for too long. Both sex and menstruation are intertwined in a web of similarly outdated societal ideals. In terms of discussion surrounding sexual pleasure, we only really see positive reinforcement directed at straight cisgender men. For example, tabloids will slut-shame anyone who isn't a straight man (most notably, women), whereas headlines often feature some sort of pun or even encouragement when a famous man is photographed shirtless or papped with a romantic interest. Another example of how society praises men but demonizes others can be found if you look at social media platforms like Instagram and their policies regarding nudity: nipples found on breasts are routinely censored, while pecs aren't.

Double standards aside, there's also a lot of pressure for sex to look and sound how it's portrayed in the media and pornography. Porn offers a fantasy, and people watch it for entertainment (Fig. 27). You probably won't see things like awkward reshuffling between positions, general clumsiness or other challenges people face — which is fine! But there's no denying some people *do* watch it to learn. Pair this with a lack of informative and positive sex education in schools and it can lead to a lot of confusion and shame. My perception of sex was definitely warped for a long time after sleeping with people who thought everything they saw in porn was real. A lot of us grow up with a very rigid idea of what sex 'should be'. Not only does this stop people from figuring out what they like (and what they dislike) and recognizing causes for concern (like pain), but it also stops people from having agency over their bodies. With some people feeling like they can't even mention the fact they're on their period, it should come as no surprise that the thought of sharing a desire to have sex during this point in the cycle makes many feel uncomfortable.

On top of all this, you very rarely see period sex discussed in a positive light or represented in any media. The only recent example I can think of is Rachel Bloom's glorious 'Period Sex' song from the TV show *Crazy Ex-Girlfriend*, and even then the full version was deemed too 'dirty' for television. Talking about *all* aspects of menstruation can help normalize these discussions and empower people to either take action or consider changing their views.

Whether you're someone who has a period or not, a penchant (or even an indifference) for period sex is totally normal and healthy. If you are someone who does feel horny while on their period and thought you were weird or alone, you are neither of these things. There's even a range of biological *and* psychological explanations that further prove just how natural this desire is. So, let's unpack them.

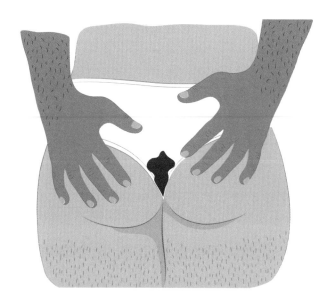

PERIOD SEX MYTHS

① YOU CAN'T GET PREGNANT DURING A PERIOD

While the possibility is small, it can still happen. Remember, sperm can live in the uterus for up to five days! If you have unprotected sex near the end of a period and there isn't a huge gap between menstruation and ovulation, it's possible sperm could still be present come ovulation time. If you aren't using long-term contraception such as the pill or an IUD in order to avoid pregnancy, use a barrier method such as an internal or external condom or a diaphragm.

② YOU DON'T HAVE TO WORRY ABOUT SEXUALLY TRANSMITTED INFECTIONS (STIS) WHEN HAVING PERIOD SEX

Wrong! STIs can be transferred through blood and fluids. No matter what time of the month it is, condoms are the safest way to prevent the spreading of infections through bodily fluids during sex. However, they don't protect you from STIs that can be spread from skin-to-skin contact such as herpes and genital warts. Dental dams (a soft plastic latex or polyurethane square) are also a good option that are typically used to cover genitals during oral sex.

③ MENSTRUAL BLOOD IS 'IMPURE' AND WILL INFECT ANYONE WHO COMES INTO CONTACT WITH IT

The only way a partner could be infected by menstrual blood is if there is already an infection present. Although there are lot of religious and spiritual practices that discourage people from having sex while on their periods, none of them stem from biological facts.

④ IF YOU DO GET PREGNANT, YOUR BABY WILL HAVE RED HAIR

Okay, so this is an ancient myth that I'm sure nobody still believes, but it's too funny not to include. In the Middle Ages, many thought ginger children were the result of people having sex while on their periods!

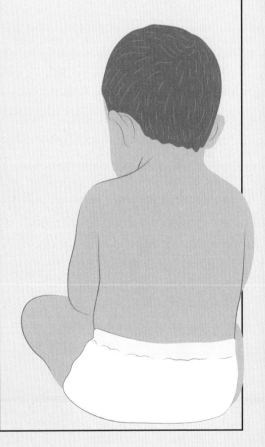

Blame It on the Hormones (Again)

Fig. 28

One of the most common explanations medical experts turn to is our favourite hormone, progesterone. In addition to all the things we've previously blamed it for, diminishing the libido is another one of its crimes. Progesterone is at its lowest during the period, which could explain why some of us become so horny. In addition, your body generally can feel more sensitive during a period, and this extends to the reproductive organs. Alisha Vitti, author and founder of period tracking app MyFLO, suggests that sensitive nerve endings could come into play and that 'it's not in your head, it's in your pelvis.' When the uterus is expanding with blood, it can press upon nerve endings in the pelvic area. All this extra pressure can stimulate the vulva, and the brain might interpret it as if something is actually touching you there. This theory certainly explains some of my random horniness, as I frequently experience vulva ache.

Another theory involves the increase of fluid. You might have heard the classic 'free lube' joke (Fig. 28), and let me tell you, it's nothing to be sniffed at. The fluids released during this time can offer extra 'natural' lubrication, which can be beneficial during sex by reducing the need for additional lube. As somebody who has suffered terribly with multiple bouts of vaginismus (a condition that affects one's ability to engage in vaginal penetration), this is definitely a huge plus for me. It makes sex easier and a whole lot more enjoyable knowing I can relax and not worry about the possibility of penetration being painful. In fact, extra lubrication was one of the top reasons among those I spoke to who were pro period sex. One story in particular that stood out was 25–year–old Amanda's: 'Usually it takes a bit of time for my body to naturally become wet enough for penetration, but when I'm menstruating I'm already lubricated and aroused.' Amanda told me about an experience she had with her current partner (T) and now ex–girlfriend (A). They were all having sex and both she and A were menstruating, and blood ended up absolutely everywhere. Amanda describes this experience as empowering not only because it felt incredibly good but because she didn't have to worry about her partners not liking it: 'We didn't just ignore the blood, or act like it was lube, we enjoyed it for what it was.'

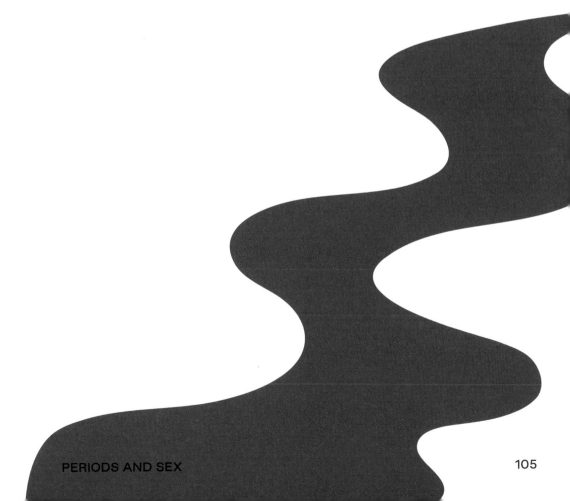

Your Brain Can Make You Horny Too

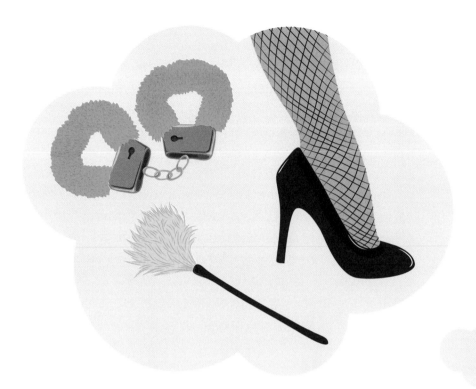

Fig. 29

Moving on to the psychological side of things, some people want sex during this time simply because they're taught not to. We're conditioned to think period sex should be forbidden, and for some this could be part of the thrill. It's human nature to want what you can't have. I felt exactly the same way when I first started having sex while I was on my period. After spending such a long time avoiding period sex, it felt truly exhilarating — and I don't just mean when I climaxed. Another mental factor that probably helps some people enjoy sex more during this time is having the risk of pregnancy significantly lowered.

Perhaps the most interesting thing of all is how arousal triggered by menstruation (and arousal in general) differs for everyone (Fig. 29). For example, I experience a desire for penetration right before my period starts and for a couple of days at the beginning of my period. Even if I don't always act on it, the urge is almost always there on these particular days. It's worth noting that penetration doesn't necessarily have to be the main or end goal, nor should it be the only way we define sex. I spoke to somebody who experiences the same heightened state of arousal, but their chosen method of relief is performing oral sex on their partner. There's a wide range of acts you can do with others, or even by yourself. I find masturbation in particular to be a really effective way to relieve tension and pain.

Having sex during a period is not only super fun, but can offer a few advantages besides extra lubrication. For example, the endor-phins released by orgasms have been known to relieve menstrual cramps depending on their strength and intensity. It is thought that climaxing can 'relax' the uterus, and the stronger the orgasm, the better it will relieve pain. In addition to this, all the contracting the uterus does during an orgasm can actually decrease the length of a period. Having an orgasm can increase the rate at which the uterine lining sheds from the body, meaning a period could shorten by a day or two. If that's not a good reason to consider period sex, I don't know what is!

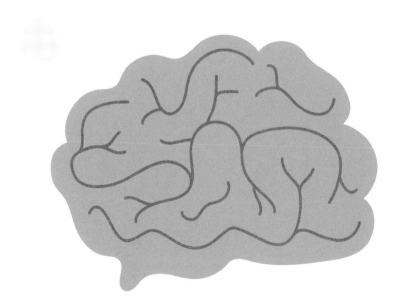

It's Okay to Dislike Period Sex

While many of these reasons explain why some of us are more aroused during this part of the menstrual cycle, they are also perfectly valid reasons as to why somebody might not enjoy period sex. For example, higher levels of progesterone can make genitals feel a little swollen and sensitive at various points in the cycle. This could add to arousal for some, or it could have the total opposite effect for others who might not want to be touched. I know sensitive genitals can either make or break a sexual encounter for me; it's either a complete no-go or it makes it easier to climax. Talk about from one extreme to the other — and I can never tell until the exact moment I'm touched. Comfort is definitely another underlying reason for apathy towards period sex. Most of the people who avoid this act do so because it doesn't make them feel good: I found that the most common reasons were lack of arousal and not feeling sexy. Siobhán, who is 35, told me that her periods can be so painful she doesn't want to be touched by anyone — even if she is engaging in sexual acts with other people: 'I will be sexual with people but I don't want anyone to touch my vulva or anything within that region. I feel really sore and tender, I just cannot face it.'

Pain is often a common denominator when it comes to periods, so it's not surprising to me that this is the reason why so many people would rather wait until their period is over. It's also not uncommon for tastes and preferences to change, as well as circumstances. I spoke to Frankie, 34, who has gone through phases of being up for period sex and of not wanting it at all. She eventually settled into feeling like it's not her thing: 'My periods aren't naturally very heavy or long but I do always have about two days where I feel really lethargic and in pain; there's a kind of heaviness in my lower body. None of this makes me feel sexy and I'd rather just take that time to regroup in my own way.' She also went on to state that there has been a noticeable drop in energy during her periods since having a baby, which means a period for her is very much a time to rest. Does the urge still arise, though? 'I do sometimes feel horny but I'd rather have a wank than be with a partner — I guess it just feels like a time to look after myself!'

Whether we just know or learn from experience, another reason many avoid period sex is simply not being able to handle blood. I spoke to a squeamish 26-year-old, Elena, who told me about a hilarious moment where she learned period sex was not for her. After having sex with a new guy she was dating, she waited until he fell asleep to remove her sea sponge. This particular form of menstrual wear does not always come with a string as a tampon does: 'After several rounds of enthusiastic banging, my sponge had been wedged in tight, slick with vaginal fluid, blood and semen. I struggled for ages to pull it out with my fingers and I spent a ridiculous amount of time trying to lever it out with a teaspoon (yes, really). In the end, I had to squat in his bathroom and basically birth the thing. Eventually it plopped out, along with all the fluids it had absorbed. To this day he still thinks that his housemate injured himself in the night and left a stain (Fig. 30).'

Fig. 30

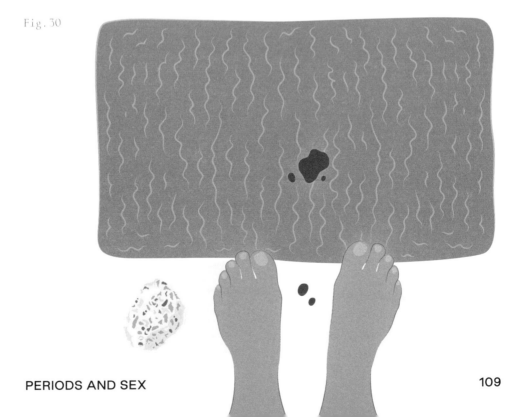

Stories like this may lead to the question, how much blood is lost during period sex? With the average amount of blood loss through–out the entirety of a period thought to be up to five tablespoons, it's probably not as much as it looks like. If sex happens towards the end of the period, there might not even be any at all! For me, it's more the gushing motion that makes it seem like it's a lot of blood. I have also found that if there are multiple stains from moving around, as opposed to one big stain, it can look like a lot. Of course bloodshed does vary, and at the end of the day it all comes down to personal thresholds and what you think constitutes a mess (however, I prom–ise you it's never as bad as you think it is). There are also some measures you can take to limit mess, which brings me to the next part of this chapter. For consenting adults, here are some period sex pointers from yours truly.

HOW TO NAVIGATE PERIOD SEX

Some supplies that might come in handy:

- Consent and open-minded partner(s)
- Protection
- A towel or blanket
- A softcup
- Something to wash sex toys with
- Underwear or clothing that makes you feel good

① ALWAYS COMMUNICATE

The first and most important step when anything is introduced during sex is communication. Whether it's a one-time thing or a regular hook-up with partner(s), just talk about it! Something that is worth thinking about is when exactly you want the discussion to take place, particularly if the thought of having this conversation makes you nervous. I recommend talking beforehand if you can: it's good to know where everyone stands. That way, nobody is caught off guard. Don't worry, it doesn't have to be a big orchestrated thing. With period sex in particular, it can be as simple as bringing it up and seeing how they react. With my current partner I simply asked if having sex while I'm bleeding would be an issue (it's not, huzzah!).

By no means does everyone have to educate their partner, but I do think it can sometimes help. If your partner is not averse to something but would like to know more, it might be worth explaining why period sex isn't dangerous or unhygienic. Perhaps you could explain why you want to do it or how it helps you. If your partner is concerned about the mess, remember that many of us don't worry about bodily functions or cleaning toys when having sex on a regular day. Sometimes it could just be a case of trying it and seeing if it's for them, but of course do not force anyone to do something they don't want to.

② TRY NOT TO JUDGE

If you don't get the answer you are hoping for, try to remind yourself that not all objections stem from sexist views. I used to have a similar knee-jerk reaction myself. Dismissing how people are feeling during this time or writing it off as an exaggeration certainly stems from this kind of mindset, but some people are just genuinely squeamish.

If somebody is entertaining the idea that one bodily fluid (like semen) is acceptable and menstrual blood isn't, by all means school them. At the end of the day, menstrual blood is simply a mixture of blood and tissue that the body no longer needs. It's not dirty, it won't hurt you and it certainly won't infect anyone who comes into contact with it. Hopefully you should be able to gauge whether or not they are objecting for no reason or genuinely concerned. After all, there is a huge difference between personal preference and entertaining a harmful stigma.

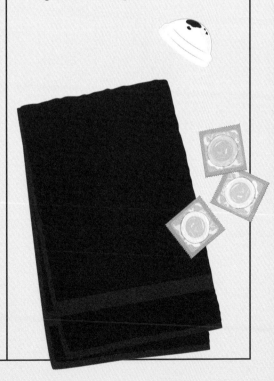

③ PREPARATION CAN SOMETIMES MAKE IT EASIER

Whether it's stocking up on supplies or figuring out your cycle, you can plan for the occasion if it helps. However, in my experience period sex does not really require a huge amount of planning. Treat it like you would any other sexual encounter, but maybe just factor in a few seconds beforehand to get the setting right if you want to avoid staining.

If it's mess-free period sex you're after, here are some other suggestions that could work:

- Use a condom if you want to do minimal clean-up afterwards
- Put a black/dark towel or blanket down wherever you are having sex, or have sex in the bath or shower and wash as you go (but please note: condoms are not effective when used in water)
- Wash sex toys as soon as you're done because dried blood can be tough to remove sometimes
- Try using a softcup (disposable) or Ziggy Cup (reusable) — both are designed to be worn during sex, as they sit close to the cervix and collect blood

Alternatively, another easy step is to just go for it and worry about the mess later. Whatever you do, stay safe and have fun!

④ DON'T LET SHAME HOLD YOU BACK

One thing that really struck a chord with me is something I was told by one of the people I spoke to. As somebody who doesn't enjoy period sex, she told me she felt like she was missing out on a vital part of being a feminist and essentially letting the team down. This only further highlights the need to change the way we discuss periods and sexual pleasure. In reality, knowing you don't want something and actively taking ownership of that is probably one of the most feminist things you can do for yourself.

Representation shouldn't just focus on the opposite ends of the spectrum. People of all ages and genders experience menstruation (and sex) differently, so why isn't this huge variety represented in the ways we discuss menstruation? We should be seeing a plethora of experiences getting equal attention. The truth is, the world doesn't have to stop for a week just because society thinks that's what people who menstruate *should* do. You can enjoy a range of activities during a period, sex included. If shame and embarrassment are the only things holding you back, consider this positive encouragement to go forth and have bloody sex!

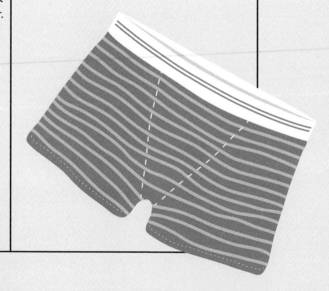

HOW BE POSI (OR

TO

PERIOD

TIVE

NEU-

TRAL)

What Is Period Positivity?

You might have heard the terms 'period positivity' or 'period positive' before and you may be thinking: 'Is that for people who are into period art, free bleeding and celebrating periods? That's not really my cup of tea; I hate mine. Does this mean I'm not period positive and therefore a bad feminist or ally?' No, not at all! While those things *are* certainly period positive, there's more to it than that. Period positivity is a particular branch of modern feminism that is often largely misunderstood and sometimes co-opted by mainstream brands as well as trans-exclusionary radical 'feminists' (TERFs — people who claim to be feminists, but are actually transphobic). It's hard to pinpoint the exact beginnings of the movement. However, UK-based comedian, writer and education researcher Chella Quint coined the phrase 'period positive' in 2006 and founded the online #periodpositive campaign (Fig. 31) to challenge taboos. It was through watching her on stage that I discovered the movement myself.

Fig. 31

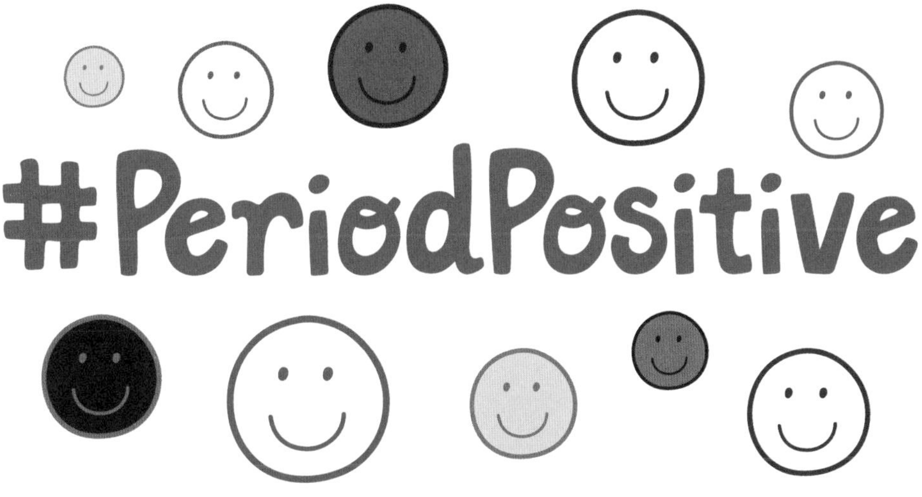

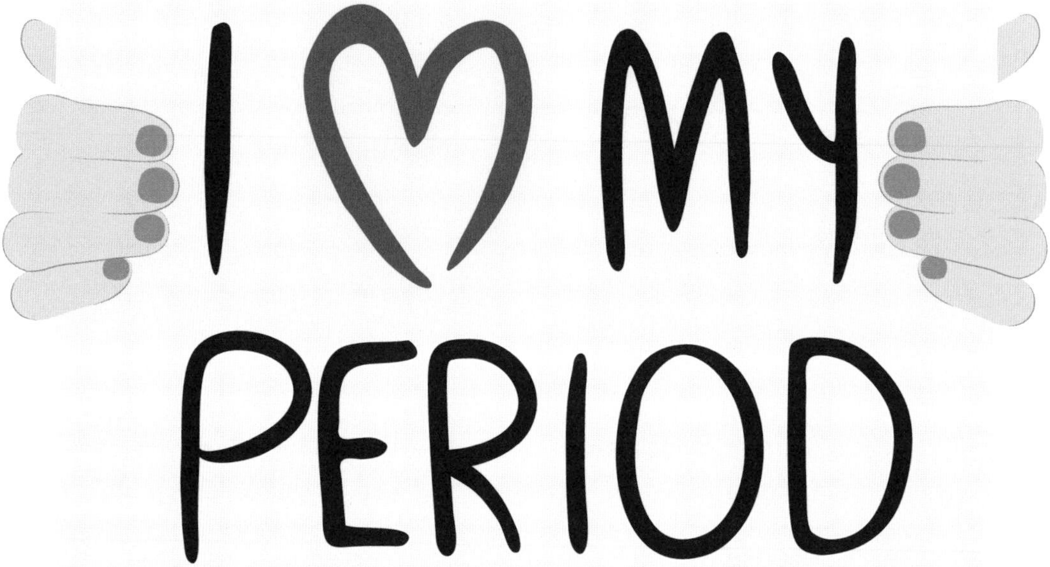
I ♥ MY
PERIOD

Do I Have to Feel Positive About My Period to Be Period Positive?

Does this mean people are wrong for expressing their feelings towards their own periods, even if they're negative? No, but language *is* important. To me, the heart of period positivity is accepting menstruation as a normal, and even healthy, process. As we've established, it is almost always treated with disgust and as if it's not part of natural biology. A huge percentage of people don't fully understand what is happening to their bodies *because* periods are treated as something that shouldn't be discussed. If we consider how much is linked to menstrual health (fertility is just one example), and just how early on we're taught periods are 'gross', it's no wonder so many people spend years failing to fill in the blanks.

While you're free to feel however you like about your own period, there's no denying that using words with negative connotations keeps this stigma alive. With so much going on in the world, it's only natural for some to question the importance of an issue that seems trivial in the grand scheme of things. While changing language might not be the main priority in comparison to other pressing issues (such as equal pay, for example), it doesn't mean we shouldn't focus on it as well. There shouldn't be a hierarchy of issues when it comes to activism. After all, people are multifaceted! So many of us don't realize the impact our words have and how language is part of a much larger problem. For example, imagine you're experiencing something you're not quite sure about and you're trying to summon the courage to seek help about it — and you hear it described as 'dirty', 'weird' or 'unnatural'. It's likely you'd put off reaching out due to embarrassment and shame, which could potentially lead to a problem going unresolved or worsening. There's a huge difference between seeing periods as an annoying aspect of one's life, and treating them as something to be embarrassed about. And it works the other way, too: a lack of discussion gives the impression that symptoms we experience, be it extremely painful or heavy periods (or sometimes both), *aren't* cause for concern, when in reality they can often be the opposite.

The way people talk about periods can be derogatory in other ways too. For example, it's common for someone to assume a person is on their period whenever they show emotion — be it sadness or anger — instead of examining their own behaviour (you could piss me off any day of my cycle; maybe you're just a prick!). Not only is the phrase 'you're just on your period' a super embarrassing cliché, it diminishes people's feelings. When you jump to this conclusion, you're telling that person they're being irrational and their feelings don't matter. If we let things like this slide, we're only reinforcing the idea that it's okay to shame people for simply being on their periods. Think about how silly that is for a minute.

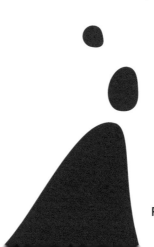

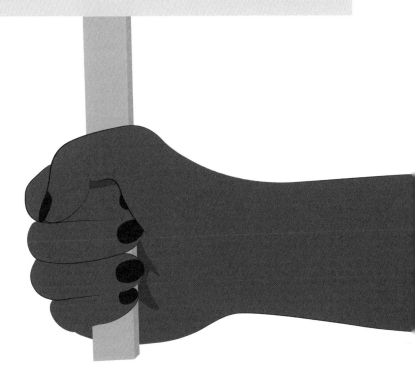

Fig. 32

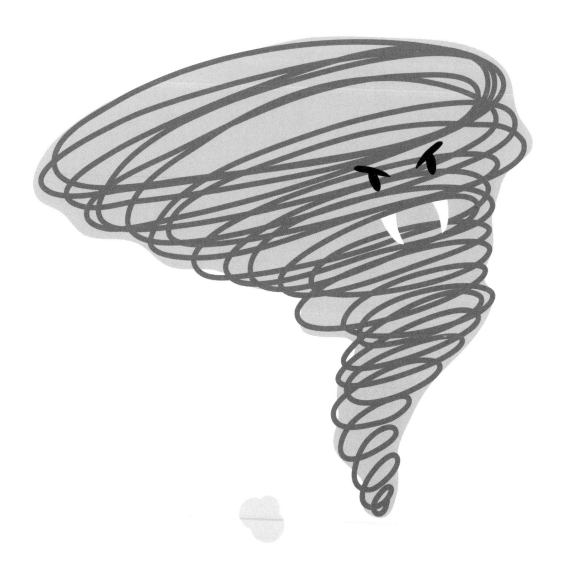

RED MOON GANG

The Cycle of Shame

Society seems to be stuck in a vicious cycle (Fig. 32) where people react childishly to even the slightest mention of periods, making those around them who menstruate feel the need to hide it. While of course you don't have to shout it from the rooftops (but also — if you want to, why not?), if people can't even utter the word 'period' then we've obviously got a problem. What makes this cycle even harder to break is just how early on it's implemented. From the moment you're old enough to understand what a period is (whether you have them or not), you often learn they are an inherently bad thing that should be hidden, and because of the insidious nature of taboos, many people treat their *own* period like this too. In turn, people who don't menstruate grow up absorbing negative ideas from each side. They can take on and project an attitude that makes menstruating folks around them feel like it's safer to suffer in silence, thus exacerbating the problem.

If those who menstruate continue to avoid freaking out their peers who don't get it, things are going to take even longer to change. Having said that, though, the onus isn't just on us. People who don't menstruate, particularly cisgender men, I am calling on you to challenge your buddies more on this outdated way of thinking. The next time you hear a silly joke, challenge it. If your friend is venting about somebody who happens to be on their period, ask them to consider the possibility they might have just upset them. If your friend is having a rough period, show some support, even if it's just listening to them vent. Reproduction affects *all* genders (remember, we wouldn't exist without it!), and so does the ignorance surrounding it. We all have the power to combat stigma.

Brands Are Just as Much to Blame

Of course, it's not just individuals reinforcing this stigma. Brands perpetuate the idea that periods should be hidden when they use words like 'discreet' (Fig. 33), and when they actively choose not to include menstrual blood, or at least red liquid, in their adverts. When discussing this online, a 29-year-old reached out with a story that has stayed with me: 'I once had a period so light, I freaked out and turned to my group chat immediately. I was so spooked and when I sent them a photo, they told me their periods looked like that all the time. I have experienced periods for about 20 years now. I have endometriosis, fibroids and have even had a chocolate cyst on my ovary. All this combined means I had never actually seen "regular" period blood because nobody shows it, or even close to it! I've had multiple surgeries because of my reproductive health and I still had no clue that this was "normal".' (This really illuminates just how much of an impact shame can have. We need to normalize every last drop of menstrual blood!).

Independent brands aren't without fault either. Many are still perpetuating inaccuracies surrounding periods, as well as the vagina, whether it's through harmful language or specific products them-selves. A recent example of this is Mensez's 'lipstick' — the brainchild of a chiropractor who encouraged people to 'glue' their vulva shut as a way to stop menstrual leaking. He believed there was a gap in the market, but this product was born out of one thing: disgust towards menstruation. Rife with ignorant and dangerous inaccuracies, as well as a fundamental misunderstanding of how the reproductive system works, the idea was that people would flush everything out when they urinate, then reseal.

I'm sure that by this point you don't need a reminder of how menstruation works and why this is a bad idea — but let's recap, because I love a good ol' rant. First of all, the labia do not completely cover the vaginal opening. They're usually slightly above and, not to mention, come in a range of shapes and sizes. In addition, vaginal muscles frequently contract. Sometimes we don't even know they're doing it! Suggesting people 'glue' their body parts shut is not only ridiculous (because it wouldn't work), it's incredibly unsafe and insanitary. Closing it up would likely create an imbalance as the vagina is a self-cleaning organ, constantly working on a mix of both good and bad bacteria. Also, this product is just another example of how people fundamentally misunderstand the vagina. You do not urinate through the vagina. You can't plug a tampon into a bladder, so what good could gluing a vulva shut do? I shudder when I think about the potential pain and other issues a product like this could cause.

Fig. 33

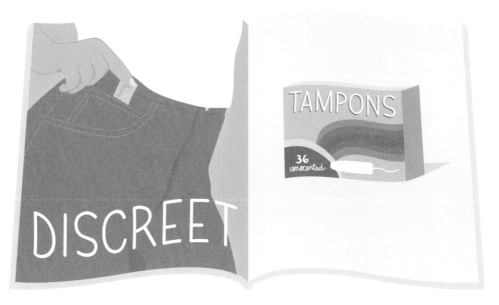

The Language of Periods

If we truly want to bring periods into the modern age, we need to adopt more inclusive language. 'Male' and 'female' are no longer the only genders people identify as today, but the words we use don't always reflect this. This issue directly relates to menstruation because not everyone who has a period is female.

A good way to get into the habit of removing gendered language as the default is to start by looking at your everyday speech. Instead of using gender-specific terms to describe professions or people, like 'fireman', opt for a more gender-neutral term such as 'firefighter'. Think about it this way: if you're already swapping terms like 'mankind' and 'history' for words that focus on women ('womankind'; 'herstory'), why not go one further and remove gender altogether?

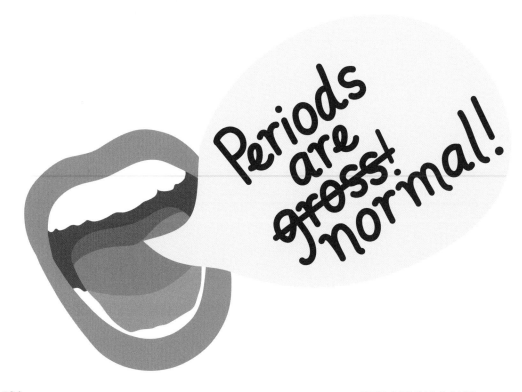

HOW GENDERED LANGUAGE AFFECTS TRANSGENDER AND NONBINARY PEOPLE

People rarely consider all the different ways in which having a period can impact someone's physical and mental wellbeing, especially since so many mental symptoms can manifest as physical ones too. Take gender dysphoria, for example. This is the term given to describe when a person experiences discomfort because their gender and the sex they were assigned at birth are not the same. This clash between sex and gender can lead to distressing feelings; a lot of things can trigger these, having a period being one of them. I spoke to hundreds of people when conducting research for this book, with nearly half being transgender and/or nonbinary. One person in particular told me that gender dysphoria for them is more than severe discomfort, it's a level of intensity that cannot be explained and essentially cuts them off from the world. They described it as dissociation with an overwhelming physical feeling.

What exactly is it abtout having a period that can cause gender dysphoria in some people? Tammy, who is nonbinary or genderqueer and 28 years old, told me that dysphoria triggered by periods can start when they walk down a shopping aisle and search for period products (Fig. 34). As Tammy leans more towards a sense of style that could be described as masculine, the thought of strangers seeing that they use what are commonly described as 'feminine hygiene products' can be incredibly overwhelming. '[A trigger for me] is generally having strangers know I'm on my period and thus classifying me as female,' they told me.

Similarly, Kai, who is 27 and masculine nonbinary, said that dysphoria has made getting a diagnosis for polycystic ovary syndrome (PCOS) very complicated: 'Doctors who understood dysphoria often suggested that this was my issue, as opposed to a "real" medical problem causing the discomfort.' Kai told me another thing people don't consider is that most medical environments, such as clinics and gynaecologists, contain posters covered with heavily gendered language that solely focuses on cisgender women. Not only does this trigger extreme discomfort, Kai also maintains that doctors with this kind of material in their practices are more likely to dismiss dysphoria. One doctor outright told Kai they were being silly when discussing how menstruation made them feel. Kai tells me that although their periods have got better over time with treatment, dysphoria still makes menstruation an incredibly hard experience to deal with: 'Pain and dysphoria feed off of one another, it's like a vicious cycle. The more stressed I am, the more pain I'm in. Period pain makes me feel more dysphoric, which makes me more stressed and so on.' They also told me that when their dysphoria is bad, it's constant — and sometimes impossible to focus on anything else.

Fig. 34

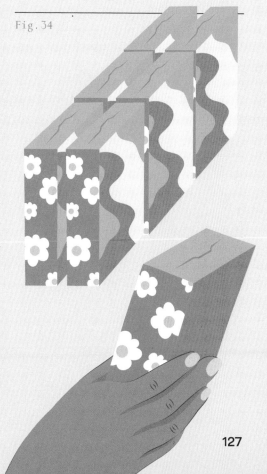

If you think about it, reducing women to their bodies is counterproductive for a number of reasons: it's what society already does and is something feminism is trying to end; it further cements transphobic ideologies; and it reinforces what a lot of transgender and nonbinary people already feel — that society doesn't respect or support them.

Two common reactions I've come across regarding the call for more inclusive language are cries of 'censorship', or the fact that it doesn't seem like a big deal. And you know, I get it. I used to have the same knee-jerk reaction myself, but it's not always about you. Yes, YOU, reading. Adapting language is not about censoring yourself, it's more about being mindful and helping everyone feel included. It's naive of us to think that language doesn't matter when it's frequently used as a tool of oppression. Furthermore, if language doesn't seem important to you then it's no biggie, right? Just swap a few words out. Celebrating the human body, especially vaginas and uteruses, which are often either sexualized or described as gross, is no doubt important. However, this can be done without excluding people who are already marginalized. Kicking somebody when they're down is not progressive or feminist, and contributes absolutely nothing to making periods less stigmatized. Language is constantly evolving and by using gender-neutral terms, we can normalize the idea that anyone can perform a job and anyone can menstruate, regardless of their gender. If true gender equality is the goal, we need to start looking at the things that perpetuate inequality — and language is one of them.

Things Are Slowly Getting Better

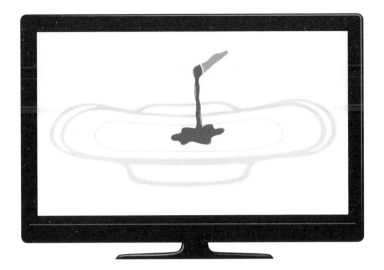

Over the years, a few brands have stepped up their advertising game. In 2017 we saw retailer Bodyform swap blue liquid for real blood (!!!) (Fig. 35) and, in 2018, Always launched their #endperiodpoverty campaign. While both of these campaigns marked a tremendous stride forward in terms of period talk becoming more mainstream, you can't help but feel a bit dubious — especially when they launched so late in the game. Often implemented or introduced when a topic is already trending, this strategy has been put in place to sell products and nothing more, thus making it seem performative. I spoke to the founder of British charity Bloody Good Period, Gabby Edlin, about this; her organization works tirelessly to eradicate the stigma surrounding menstruation and provide essential products to asylum seekers in and around London and Leeds. With a team of 200+ volunteers (and a waiting list of 500) who donate on average 100 hours a month, they've grown from providing to two North London drop-in centres to 25 projects where they send out over 6,000 products a month. Access to period products and safe, hygienic spaces in which to use them without shame or stigma is essential for anyone who menstruates. It's also a pressing issue more corporations should be focusing on. Gabby explained she finds the co-opting of the period poverty movement shocking: 'It's only been in the last few years, in response to activism, that brands have started to clean up their own acts. Hijacking the work of activists and attempting to gloss over the issue with a small amount of products will do nothing but perpetuate the problem.'

Realistically, if these corporations *really* wanted to help end period poverty, there are a range of actions they could take. For example, why not lower prices or use their power to try to encourage governments to drop the tampon tax once and for all? Let's not forget that many of these brands are partly to blame for perpetuating the stigma around periods to begin with through marketing (for example, the underlying idea that we won't be clean unless we rid ourselves of the dirty shame of menstruating by using their products). What else can these brands do? Edlin suggests, 'I would like to see brands take a real responsibility in terms of the chemicals they use and the non-environmentally-friendly products they produce, as well as responsible consultation and research-led approaches to solving the problem — alongside people already doing this work.'

For every product that misses the mark, there's often a fantastic, innovative (and often reusable) one right around the corner. What's so great about some of the independent brands and charities out there is how often they try to help. Besides encouraging and educating people when it comes to inclusive language and creating alternative products, many donate generously to people in need. For example, Ruby Cup has a 'Buy One, Give One' scheme where they donate a whole product for every purchase, as opposed to one pad per pack. In recent years, there have been products inspired by the awareness of the harm plastic does to our planet, too. For instance, UK-based startup DAME introduced their reusable tampon applicator, D, in early 2019 after completing a very successful crowdfunding campaign. Their applicator is a game-changing device designed to make periods more eco-friendly even if you use tampons, which isn't something we see often. Helping out doesn't have to be an all-or-nothing situation, and we should hope to see more of this behaviour from the industry.

But it's not just companies who are making things better. More and more, individuals are taking it upon themselves to combat period stigma in new and exciting ways. Take Daniela Gilsanz, one of the founders of a menstruation–themed board game called The Period Game. Created to inspire people to see periods as a fun, positive learning experience as opposed to an uneasy situation, the game is designed so that you can't participate without saying words like 'period', 'tampon' or 'menstrual cup'. The idea behind this is that if you can ask a friend for a pad in the game, you'll feel comfortable doing so in real life. This is a brilliantly simple way of encouraging people to talk about periods — and it's working. Gilsanz told me, 'We've played The Period Game with over 200 students as well as health educators, gynaecologists and child psychologists to ensure that it is as fun and informative as possible. In playing the game with young people we've heard so many different period stories and had the fortune of seeing people shout, "I want my period!" at the top of their lungs.'

Normalizing such discussions really does stir up tremendous support, and Gilsanz has experienced this at first hand: 'We had an 8th grader understand what PMS was for the first time, to extreme relief that she wasn't alone.' Gilsanz believes the game is capable of creating more understanding, and therefore it can help equip society to tackle the topic of period equity (meaning, making sure everyone has access to period care). The game was successfully funded via Kickstarter, which makes me excited to see what other innovative, period positive ways we can use to teach people that menstruation is nothing to be scared of.

How Else Can I Be Period Positive?

A great way we can strive to a live a more period positive life is by actively challenging ourselves to be less afraid to talk about menstruation. Check yourself when you project embarrassment onto others. Instead of shaming people for oversharing, look within and really ask yourself *why* you're reacting a certain way. Personally, a lot of my opinions and reactions used to stem from internalized misogyny. We all absorb sexist societal beliefs that demean anyone who deviates from the default (which is often white and cisgender), day in and day out. Many of us, after observing gender bias and misogynistic ideologies, apply them to ourselves and others around us — often unknowingly. For example, after experiencing a former partner reacting badly to a surprise period, I carried that disgust with me for many years. Every time the topic of menstruation arose, I was instantly pulled back to that moment and felt ashamed. It's worth taking the time to acknowledge your own personal bias and trying to pinpoint where it comes from. Not everything can be blamed on other people's beliefs of course, but the next time you judge somebody for speaking about periods, ask yourself: how does this personally affect me? Once you rid yourself of shame and stigma, continue to break the cycle and make a point of speaking about menstruation more openly. Talk to your friends about it and share period stories, inform the non-menstruating folks in your life about the process or express when you're feeling rough, challenge ignorance and bigotry when you can, teach your kids about it so they can grow up with a healthy attitude, and so on.

Another way in which the period positive movement helps people to view menstruation in a less negative light is through encouraging them to engage in self-care around this time. Menstrual awareness is becoming an increasingly popular part of the wellness umbrella (Fig. 36), leading to a rise in menstrual health, fertility and hormone coaches. Although these coaches focus on different top-ics, an ethos that is shared is seeing periods as a sacred time of sorts. Think of your period as a metaphor. Given that this is a time where the uterus is quite literally shedding or letting go, the idea is that menstruation is a good time to see what else you need to shed. What is no longer serving you? Channel your inner Marie Kondo and get rid of anything that doesn't spark joy!

Something I like to do is take note of things that have annoyed me over the course of the month and see if there's a pattern. Am I easily irritated at certain points of my cycle? (Yes.) Can I avoid this

Fig. 36

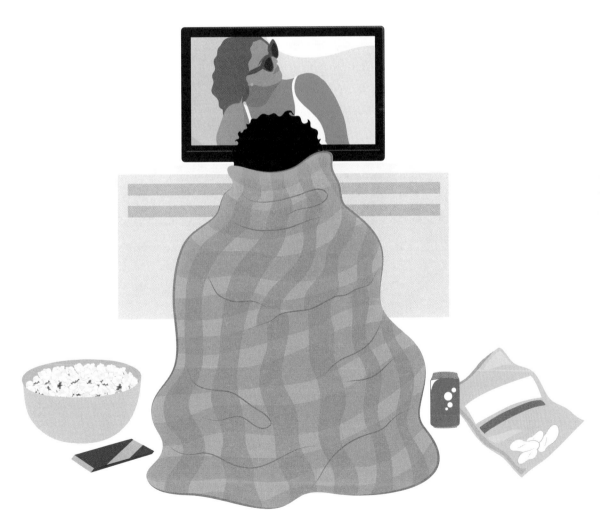

at all? (Maybe.) Since emotions are heightened for me during my period, embracing the fact that I'm feeling everything about 500 times harder has allowed me to understand my reactions more. A period offers an opportunity to find out more about yourself; it allows you to explore *why* you respond to things in a certain way. Failing that, there's never a more appropriate time for a good, cathartic cry, if you ask me.

Periods can help you practise being kinder to your body, too. Try to rid yourself of the guilt that can sometimes come with craving certain foods. Don't beat yourself up if a certain product isn't compatible with your body (sometimes I can't get my cup inside me, despite having years of experience). Avoid consuming media that lists all the things you *should* be doing while menstruating, like exercising. If this does help you, cool! On the other hand, if you just want to have a lie down, that's totally fine too. Period positivity encourages you to set your own personal boundaries. If a period is a time that triggers negative feelings, allow yourself to feel bad and own that. If you generally view your period as a positive thing but you're just not into it one month, I understand. If the feeling is neutral, that's also OK. For me, it's all about trying to be less hard on myself and accepting that my feelings can change at any point.

→ Period positivity is freedom to communicate how bad your period is.
→ Period positivity is advocating for cheaper, or even free, menstrual products.
→ Period positivity is protesting the tampon tax.
→ Period positivity is calling for menstrual equity.
→ Period positivity is using more inclusive language.
→ Period positivity is calling for healthcare providers to take pain more seriously.
→ Period positivity is calling out people who dismiss valid concerns or feelings.
→ Period positivity is no longer entertaining offensive jokes.
→ Period positivity is listening to people who menstruate.
→ Period positivity is stocking public bathrooms with free period products.

→ Period positivity is making art with menstrual blood or art that makes a statement.

→ Period positivity is whatever you want it to be.

While adopting inclusive language is a good first step, it doesn't mean you have to change the way you view your own period (unless you want to!). If you hate your period, I totally get that. Hell, you can even be period neutral if you like. Nobody is asking you to change your mind or trying to invalidate your experiences; in fact, the period positive movement encourages the freedom to express just how bad your period makes you feel.

All this sounds pretty straightforward, right? Instead of focusing on simple tasks that — when done by the masses — could have great momentum, the period positivity movement is often reduced to a stereotype of extreme and unreasonable people who just want to bleed everywhere. Think of the impact some of these tasks could have if everyone did their bit: me, you, employers, the government, everyone. This movement is not about policing how individuals feel about their periods, it's about challenging long-held unfair perceptions of menstruation as a whole. What kind of message are we sending when we use words and phrases like 'discreet', 'gross', 'feminine hygiene' and 'disgusting'? You can express your ambivalence towards your own period without perpetuating the myth that menstruation is something to be ashamed of. You can discuss a bodily function without alienating a part of the population. And, most importantly, it's never too late to make that change.

Small Period Positive Steps
You Can Take Every Day

→ Stop censoring yourself and speak about periods openly
→ Try not to project embarrassment onto others
→ #livetweetyourperiod
→ Actively talk about your periods with your family and friends
→ Carry period products around with you
→ Stop hiding your products when you go to the bathroom
→ Shop with brands that try to combat period poverty
→ Wear something that makes a statement (Fig. 37)
→ Adapt your language and be more inclusive

Fig. 37

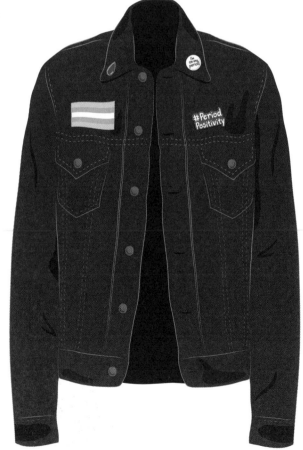

AROUND

IN 30

THE
WORLD

PERIODS

Periods Are Viewed Differently Across the Globe

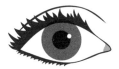 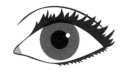

By this point I think we can agree that the body's monthly(ish) visitor is a pretty natural part of life. But no matter how many times this visitor unexpectedly turns up, periods remain taboo across the globe. Although there's no shortage of things we can blame this on, there is no denying that tradition and a lack of education are two of the biggest factors. Undoing years of harmful practice is no small feat. When an act as simple as telling someone your period has arrived is still frowned upon, what impact does it have and how does one break the cycle of misinformation? Let's explore how period stigma affects people globally and the incredible activists working to solve this societal problem.

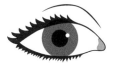 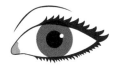

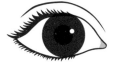 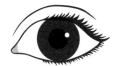

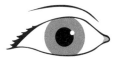 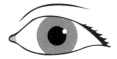

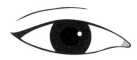 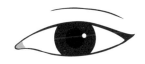

You Could Be Banished to a Hut

If people know you're on your period in certain parts of Nepal and India, you may be forced to bleed it out in a hut (Fig. 38). In Nepal, the beliefs behind this practice — called *Chhaupadi* — stem from Hinduism and dictate what somebody on their period can do, what they can eat, when they can sleep and whom they can interact with. These sheds are often dark, unhygienic and unbearable in any weather, not to mention riddled with insects, dung and whatever muck animals bring in. If cattle sheds are not available, a makeshift hut is used instead.

Although this custom was outlawed by Nepal's supreme court in 2005, the practice is still very much in place. Radha Paudel, head of organization Action Works Nepal (AWON), says this tradition is so instilled that, when abroad, some Nepalese people still practise it. She also told *The Guardian* that, in places where land is too expensive, people will still live separately during their periods — even if the family rents only a single room. This tradition has been linked to psychological and physical illnesses, danger of attack from both people and wild animals, as well as the possibility of death.

Huts in India are known as *gaokors*. In the part of the world where the practice occurs they don't allow those who are menstruating to cook, even if they're alone. Instead, the hut's occupants rely on family to bring food and other items, sometimes as far as to the edge of the forest. Many are forced to live in isolation for one week a month and, since the *gaokors* are considered public property, nobody maintains them — so when it rains, it pours. Water often finds a way in, and roofs leak. In 2015, the NGO Society for Peoples Action in Rural Services and Health (SPARSH) visited 223 *gaokors* in tribal areas and found that 98 per cent of them were missing proper beds, let alone electricity and other basic amenities. A thick sheet is often used in place of a mattress, and this doubles up as a cushion during the daytime. They also found that the majority of the inhabitants of these huts create makeshift bathrooms out of bamboo. In addition, with the huts being so far away, many people have died from injuries from wild animals, like snake bites, while staying there. The custom of sending people to huts is so ingrained in India that local self-governing bodies work towards bringing huts closer to the village — instead of trying to eradicate the practice altogether.

Fig. 38

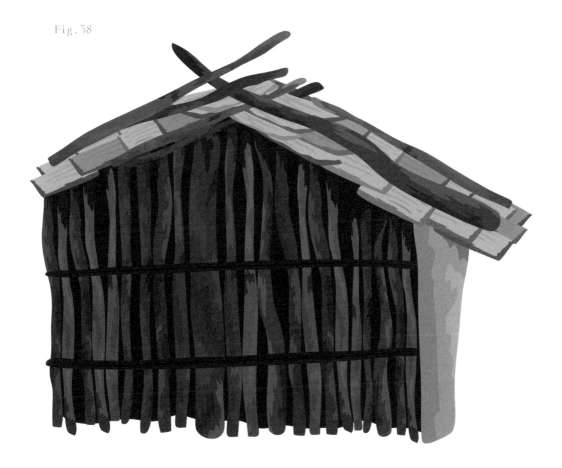

Inaccurate Myths are Still in Place

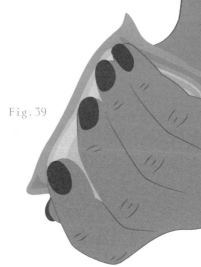

Misinformation is unfortunately still being taken as Fig. 39 gospel all around the world. For example, from a young age, some people in Afghanistan are told to avoid showering during menstruation. This inaccurate belief stems from a fear that people will become infertile if they do so, and the no-showering rule also extends to washing genitals.

Another disturbing and isolating myth comes from Bolivia. In certain parts of the country, people are encouraged to keep their pads completely hidden at all times (Fig. 39). If you're someone who prefers discretion, this might not sound so bad. However, since menstrual hygiene is not part of the school curriculum there, many believe they are inflicted with a terrible disease. This fear is so instilled in people that they think menstrual blood has the power to carry sickness or long-term illnesses like cancer, and contaminates other waste in bins. Of course, there is not an ounce of truth to this — but even teachers reinforce it. Although there are designated areas where one can dispose of pads, many don't feel comfortable enough to use them. Instead, people opt for carrying used pads around until they can throw them away at home. A few years ago, the children's charity UNICEF investigated around 10 schools in Bolivia. They concluded that one of the main challenges faced by those who menstruate is limited access to private bathrooms and the shame this brings.

You Might Not Be Allowed Near Food

It's not just waste bins or their own bodies that menstruating folk supposedly pollute. In parts of both India and Africa, many are convinced that those with period blood exiting their bodies will spoil food if they so much as touch it. The most fascinating, and perhaps most distressing, aspect of these misconceptions is how they can differ depending on geographical region. Generally, in countries where these beliefs are held, people are told to avoid cooking altogether. However, in some areas of Zambia, food restrictions are even more specific: not only are you forbidden from cooking while on your period, you can't add salt to your meal either (Fig. 40).

Developing countries are not the only places where these types of beliefs are entertained. Every day, insidious practices are enforced in curious ways across the globe. In parts of Japan, people believe that menstruation causes an 'imbalance' in taste, leaving those with periods excluded from the sushi industry (Fig. 41) as it is thought they cannot have a reliable taste in food. Is there any truth to this? As we've said, PMS symptoms can sometimes have an effect on factors like hunger levels or cravings (whether there's an increase or decrease), but does this mean they would affect one's ability to be a sushi chef? In 2015 Vilma Blondet de Azeredo, associate professor at a Brazilian nutrition school, and her colleagues conducted a study which explored exactly this. Looking into the influence of the menstrual cycle on taste and food intake, fifty people of 'childbearing age' (which in the medical industry typically means cisgender women aged 20 to 35) were followed for three months. They concluded that the menstrual cycle can change acid taste perception, which affects food choices in the luteal phase (post-ovulation, pre-period). This suggests that hormones such as insulin and ghrelin (the hunger hormone) can influence taste perception, which controls food intake.

While fruit is the food group most commonly associated with acidic taste, dairy products, fish and fresh meat also come under this category — all food commonly found in popular sushi dishes.

While there may be *some* scientific truth behind this practice, I can't imagine it to be so serious an issue that it warrants a gender gap. Speaking from personal experience, I have never noticed a massive change in taste when I'm menstruating other than certain foods really hitting the spot. I am neither a chef nor a sushi expert, but surely recipes and guidelines would be followed and your food would be checked if this really was a concern.

In addition, did you know that Japan became the first country in the world to grant menstrual leave back in 1947? This is a type of leave where people who menstruate have the option to take paid (or in some cases, unpaid) leave from employment when they're on their period and unable to go to work because of it. This hasn't quite taken off worldwide yet, but a few countries implement it. In Japan, the law was put in place mainly because people believed work was too injurious to health during menstruation. So, surely the people who are apparently unable to make good sushi while menstruating wouldn't necessarily be at work and making sushi during this time anyway? Also, newsflash, this part of the population you're excluding eats sushi too!

Figs 40–41

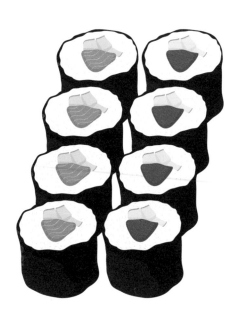

Periods Are Simply Not Discussed

The cycle of poverty in developing countries plays a big part in why menstruation is still so taboo there. In Malawi, one of the most impoverished countries on earth, periods are simply not discussed. Here in particular, around 85 per cent of the population live in rural areas, meaning education is unaffordable in remote communities. Access to financial services is restricted; many are without jobs and have very little money. A lot of Malawians work in agriculture, but it's hard to produce enough crops to maintain substantial income. Further to this, they face a number of other obstacles on a daily basis. When people fall ill, there's not enough money to treat the problem well. People are forced to miss out on education because they cannot afford period products. About 30 per cent of children in Malawi do not start primary school, even though it is free. Many choose to drop out, as dealing with the embarrassment of not being prepared for their period is too much to bear.

In Korea, at the time of writing, there is barely any representation at all. You'll find virtually no adverts for period products, as pads must be hidden from men at all times – even from husbands at home. Menstruation *did* make the headlines in 2017 when toxins were discovered in products from a major supplier. Thousands took legal action after suffering negative effects such as skin rashes and painful cramps after using Lilian brand pads and products by Clean Nara. One of the women seeking compensation from the brand told the *Korea Herald* that she believed the problem is not confined to the Lilian pad: 'I cannot believe that the government had the Lilian pad pass its standards. I don't think any brand is safe to use.' This started a dialogue about the lack of conversation surrounding periods, and the lack of transparency from companies when it comes to products in particular.

The Tampon Tax Is Still a Thing

In many parts of the world, period products (most notably tampons) are taxed as non-essential 'luxury' items. Because bleeding heavily for days on end *screams* luxurious, right? Although there have been a number of efforts to push governments to scrap this tax altogether, only a handful of countries have followed through, or at least made a start. The French parliament voted to lower the tax from a whopping 20 per cent to 5.5 per cent in 2015, and the UK scrapped it altogether in the 2020 Budget. (For comparison, in Italy, the tampon tax is even higher at 22 per cent.) During the same year, Canadian politician Irene Mathyssen led a successful campaign that saw Canada scrap its national goods and service tax on period products altogether. Following years of petitions from campaigners (one of which gathered nearly 200,000 signatures), Germany eliminated its tampon tax following a landmark vote in the German Parliament at the end of 2019. They were previously put into the 19 per cent tax bracket, the highest tax rate possible in the European country, making these products subject to some of the highest taxes on period products of any country in the European Union.

The same can't be said for America, though, where at the time of writing only 18 out of 50 states are without the tampon tax (Fig. 42). Between 1975 and 2005, a mere five states got rid of it. Massachusetts was one of the first to drop the tax, alongside Minnesota, Pennsylvania, New Jersey and Maryland. Since then a further eight have followed suit: New York, Florida, Illinois, Connecticut, Nevada, Utah, Rhode Island and Ohio. New York scrapped the tax in July 2016 after Governor Andrew Cuomo described it as 'a regressive tax on essential products' and signed legislation eliminating local and state sales taxes on period products. For people living in Delaware, Oregon, Montana, New Hampshire and Alaska, the tampon tax is not an issue, as these states do not have sales tax in general. This leaves 32 states out of 50 that still implement the tampon tax. Former US president Barack Obama addressed this issue in an interview with YouTuber Ingrid Nilsen back in January 2016: 'I have no idea why states would tax these as luxury items,' he said. 'I suspect it's because [cisgender] men were making the laws when those taxes were passed.'

Although Ireland is within the European Union, it's a unique case as it has no VAT on tampons, pads or panty liners. This is simply down to the fact that the 0 per cent rate was in place before the EU introduced minimum rates. A little-known fact is that it was actually countries on other continents that got the ball rolling on eliminating the tax, with Kenya being the first — there, sales tax was abolished on period products in 2004. They also ended an import duty on pads in 2011, which helped those with low incomes cut costs. A few other countries that do not enforce VAT on these items include Jamaica, Nicaragua, Nigeria, Tanzania and Lebanon. Mauritius said goodbye to their 15 per cent tax in 2017 as well.

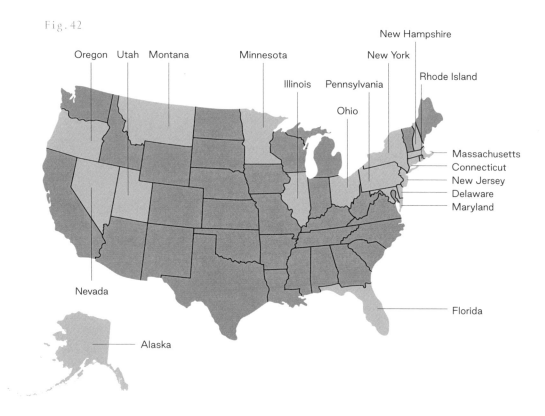

Fig. 42

Oregon Utah Montana Minnesota New Hampshire New York Rhode Island Illinois Pennsylvania Ohio Massachusetts Connecticut New Jersey Delaware Maryland Nevada Florida Alaska

Silence Harms People in Different Ways

We often forget that a lack of access to period products and bath-rooms is an obstacle for homeless people, many of whom are forced to choose between food and a box of tampons that probably won't last an entire cycle. Homeless people face large sanitary risks, too. As part of their NSFWomen series, online magazine *Bustle* inter-viewed a number of people about how they deal with their period on the street. The people in the documentary listed all the things they've been forced to use in place of period products, including napkins from restaurants, plastic bags, socks and old clothing. At one point, one of the subjects talked the audience through her washing routine. After obtaining a large drink cup from McDonalds and filling it with water, she straddles the toilet, cleaning herself with soap and using the water from the cup to rinse.

Since there are varying levels of homelessness, people struggle in different ways. For example, those who don't live in shelters have even less access to bathrooms and are at a greater risk of contracting TSS, more so if they are using makeshift tampons. Many put forward the case for reusables when trying to combat this issue, but again, this poses the risk of infection without reliable access to a bathroom. It's not just this challenge they have to deal with: people often look down on or report homeless people in public spaces. Can you imag-ine how demoralizing it is trying to find a public bathroom and then having to deal with people harassing you *on top of* bleeding?

WHAT ABOUT DISABLED PEOPLE?
By Shona Louise

There are many ways in which disabled people are left out of the conversation. We're regularly missing from supposedly diverse ad campaigns and often excluded from people's activism altogether. Our access needs are not considered and our voices almost always go unheard.

A lack of representation isn't all disabled people have to battle with, as incorrect assumptions can be just as damaging. People assume we are completely incapable; that we shouldn't be out of our homes on our own. When it comes to reproductive health in particular, I have found that the overwhelming amount of ignorance surrounding disabled people often hinders us from easily accessing healthcare. If recent efforts to ban plastic straws have taught us anything, it's that the needs of disabled people are routinely ignored. Disposable plastic straws and assistive devices that are vital to many disabled people's lives are disregarded, and the same can be said for disposable pads and tampons. Some people assume that because they can make a change, everyone else can too. Cost, mobility difficulties and chronic illnesses are just a few reasons why some of these simple changes aren't always possible.

When it comes to periods, I've found mine difficult to manage alongside my disability. I would love (and have tried) to use reusables, but re-washing — paired with the cost — doesn't work in relation to my health. As I experience chronic pain and fatigue, there are times when I have been stuck in bed, making it difficult to change pads regularly. It's easier to stick to disposable products as they require far less energy. Sometimes, as much as I want to make better choices for the environment, it just isn't possible.

Another way disabled people are excluded is through restricted access. Online, disabled people continue to share all the obstacles they face when trying to attend vital appointments like cervical screenings. In the UK where I live, NHS services have been unable to provide the hoists and postural support that some wheelchair users require. Most of us find the thought of having a cervical screening daunting, but the prospect is even more terrifying for me simply because of my access needs. Will my painful joints make it difficult? Will the room be big enough for my powerchair? The messages we keep seeing about cervical screenings have an emphasis on the importance of not delaying, and while this is a vital message, it is not an inclusive one. It doesn't end here: many have reported barriers when it comes to contraception too, as medical staff wrongly assume disabled people cannot have sex.

When facing criticism, many will argue that there is a lack of a market for products geared towards disabled people, but this could not be further from the truth. The spending power of disabled households, often referred to as the Purple Pound, was £249 billion in 2014 and 2015 in the UK alone. In the US, it was estimated at $490 billion in 2018. Globally, it's expected to exceed $8 trillion. Businesses in the UK are reportedly losing around £2 billion a month due to a lack of accessibility, something known as the Walkaway Pound. Although statistics like this are few and far between, there's an undeniable gap in the market.

So, how can we be included? First, assess the way you view disabled people. Ignoring the fact that we experience normal bodily functions like periods or engage in sexual activity causes great damage to both our mental and physical health. It blocks us from attending essential appointments. Talk to us, ask us what we need and want, stop making assumptions about our lives and experiences. Being disabled can be a full-time job: there's always a prescription that needs collecting or an appointment to attend. Just getting out of bed and dressed can take hours sometimes, so we need your help when it comes to activism. Do not speak for us, but do speak to us. Push for inclusion; if our voice is missing from a conversation, flag this. Simple acts like sharing our content online helps lift our experiences up. Ignorance surrounding disability often stems from a lack of knowledge, so signal boosting helps. One in four people are disabled, which means most people know someone who is disabled — and yet our voices still go unheard. Strive to change that.

Shona Louise is a writer and disabled activist who lives in the UK. She has written for and worked with The Guardian, Metro and Channel 4 and has been running a blog since 2011. She primarily focuses on topics such as accessibility and ableism, as well as raising awareness of disabled people's needs.

RED MOON GANG

Let's not forget about those who are incarcerated, either. An extremely small number of low-quality pads are provided to inmates (assuming the prison provides them at all). Better than nothing, right? Not when people are forced to wear a single pad for days on end. Former inmate Chandra Bozelko told *The Guardian* in 2015, 'I have seen pads fly right out of an inmate's pants. Prison maxi pads don't have wings and they have only average adhesive so, when a woman wears the same pad for several days because she can't find a fresh one, that pad often fails to stick to her underwear and the pad falls out.' While pads are often available for sale to prisoners, many can't afford them.

Think about how many period products you go through in a day. A running theme with all of these issues is the humiliation not being able to afford protection brings. Most of us have feared the possibility of bleeding through (or worse, experienced it) — and it happens on a regular basis in prisons, making the already powerless feel more dehumanized. Menstruation is an experience that degrades inmates, Bozelko writes: 'Prison makes us hate a part of ourselves; it turns us against our own bodies.' With reusables not being the appropriate solution in all situations, it's circumstances like this that make the case for free disposable products even stronger.

Why Focus on Stigma?

With traditions and beliefs like this still firmly in place and continuing to perpetuate taboos surrounding menstruation, the link between stigma and period poverty (namely, access to products) is undeniable. For example, a 2016 study led by the Department of Clinical Sciences at Liverpool School of Tropical Medicine and involving nearly 100,000 people in India found that almost half of them a) did not learn about what a period was until they experienced it for the first time, and b) thought they were dying or had a disease, as they did not know what was causing the pain and blood.

Without proper education (Fig. 43), misconceptions will continue to alienate thousands of already vulnerable people. Being shamed for having a period is distressing enough as it is, but it's even more intense when so many parts of your life are put on pause. A lack of open discussion leaves people confused and worried, and forces them to use whatever they can find in place of period products. In developing countries in particular this could mean anything from old rags to socks or newspapers, twigs, leaves or plastic bags. If your first thought is something along the lines of 'but how would that work?', that's not the takeaway here. The point is, people are left with no choice but to use literally anything they can get their hands on inconspicuously. Some like to argue that menstrual products are cheaper than alternatives like socks, but that isn't the case for those who live in poverty or are without access to shops or money. In certain places, even the cheapest kind of pad can be too expensive and many are forced to fashion some form of protection from the items that *are* available to them.

The stigma that surrounds periods directly affects people's futures, too. Not only does it make a natural bodily function an incredibly isolating experience, it also holds people who menstruate back from education and access to jobs. According to Plan International UK, 1 in 10 people who menstruate cannot afford to buy period products. In 2017, *The London Economic* reported that over 137,700 children in the UK had missed school because of this. A child who skips school every time they menstruate will receive approximately 145 fewer days of education than somebody who doesn't have periods. This is why it's so important that campaigns which push for free products also focus on destigmatizing periods.

Fig. 43

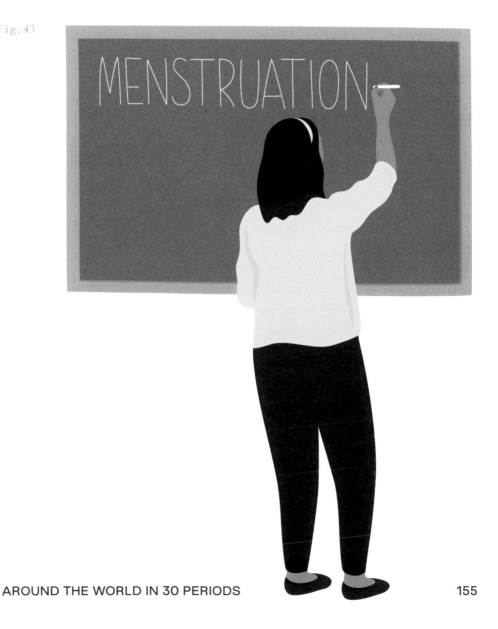

People Are Working Towards Change

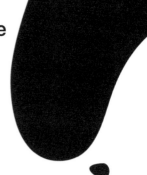

Fortunately, there is an abundance of people working to eradicate both stigma and poverty in creative ways. For example, Yuki Chizui decided to directly combat Japan's gender inequality in the food industry by opening the country's first women-run sushi restaurant in 2010. More recently, in 2019, Manjit Gill from the charity Binti International realized that many of the taboos rife in countries like India also exist within the UK. She decided to take action and get temples involved; as a result, the Shepherd's Bush Gurdwara (temple) has become the first in the world to launch a period policy. This focuses on eliminating restrictions for people during their periods by providing free products and running workshops on menstrual health. Gill told *Glamour UK* that, since launching the policy, she has been contacted by temples around the world asking her to help set up similar projects.

When looking to help combat period poverty, many activists choose to focus on youth, such as Sandhya Chaulagain of WaterAid Nepal. Since traditions are typically upheld by older people, those who believe religion shouldn't be questioned, or those who simply know no different, focusing on making things better for young people allows this charity to reach future elders who could potentially be change-makers in their communities. Using the idea that the first step to implementing appropriate menstrual care is to start at the top and educate role models better, the organization teaches men and traditional healers about debunking inaccurate myths related to periods.

There are also organizations focused on helping people who are directly impacted. Take Evelien Post and her social enterprise Supreme Reusable Sanitary Pads, for example. They are not only creating products for people in rural Malawi to use, but are helping these individuals to provide for themselves and their families. Post told me that the idea for this venture started when she first visited Malawi representing a foundation she was working for at the time. There, she discovered that most of the schoolchildren didn't know what period products were — they were using old cloths instead, which caused friction and blisters on their legs. After finding this lack of access unacceptable, she started to work on a solution. With an initial pad design already tested thanks to her predecessors at the foundation, Post quickly transformed it into the social enterprise it is today.

Menstruating in a country as poor as Malawi is a struggle simply because many don't have enough money to eat, let alone buy pads (which cost more than some people can make in a day). Supreme has five full-time and two part-time Malawian employees, and all materials they use are purchased within the country. These employees directly benefit, as they no longer have to rely on their partners for money. In addition to tailoring pads, Supreme encourages their staff to go into education should they choose to. After being taught about menstrual hygiene and presentation skills, they can host informative sessions in schools and health centres. Here, they can spread the word about the benefits of reusable pads and the importance of appropriate menstrual care. One of Supreme's employees is 24 years old and never finished secondary school; she is now in an adult learner's programme and Supreme are supporting her all the way to her diploma. This newfound independence, along with a contemporary set of skills, will benefit the employees enormously for the rest of their lives. All of these are great examples of how alternatives to classic ways of providing aid can help overall poverty.

When it comes to issues such as the tampon tax, petitions aren't the only way to take action. If anything positive has come from the tax refusing to budge, it's the new and creative ways in which people are channelling their anger. In 2017 I spoke to the founder of an Australian synchronized swimming team called The Clams. Armed with tampon-shaped pool floats (Fig. 44), this water ballet ensemble is owning periods by refusing to be embarrassed by them and raising money for those who cannot afford sanitary items. They have continued to make crimson waves on social media, raising awareness of other taboo topics like body hair. In 2018, Australia finally saw a positive end to an 18-year campaign to make period products exempt from a nationwide goods and service tax. We have campaigners dedicated to raising awareness by simply starting a discussion — as The Clams do — to thank for this landmark vote.

Fig. 44

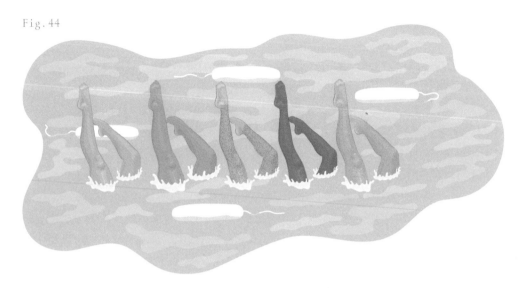

Events are another great way to effectively open a dialogue, which is exactly what 21-year-old activist Nadya Okamoto did with PERIOD CON conferences. Not only does her organization distribute period products (both reusable and disposable) to people in need, it also actively encourages youth leaders at universities and high schools around the United States to get involved. Their focus is working towards social and legal change surrounding equal access to products and, at PERIOD CON, people are encouraged to learn more about the fight for menstrual equity. With panel discussions and seminars, Okamoto hopes people leave feeling empowered, inspired and equipped with the tools they need to take action in their communities. If you're unable to attend such events, Okamoto advises that everyone can 'just start talking about periods as a normal, natural biological function. Start conversations, talk about the need to get rid of the stigma, talk about why we need to eradicate period poverty — and then take action.'

Other memorable ways people have directly responded to politicians and helped start conversations around period poverty include:

- Activists Charlie Edge and Ruth Howard donning fake blood on their white trousers outside the Houses of Parliament in London
- Project Period's Tampon Taxi that distributed menstrual products to homeless shelters around London (Fig. 45)
- The website Pornhub encouraging their menstruating users to enjoy a free week of ad-free pornography to promote orgasms as a way to alleviate period pain
- Artist Sarah Levy using her menstrual blood to create a portrait of Donald Trump after he made sexist remarks towards journalist Megyn Kelly, and auctioning the piece off to raise money for an immigrants' rights organization
- Musician Kiran Gandhi running the London marathon without a tampon to raise awareness for those who don't have access to them

These bold, fascinating ways to start a very important discussion are proof that activism works. In 2019 alone we saw *Period. End of Sentence.*, a documentary film about menstruation in India, win an Oscar, the release of a period emoji, and periods become a part of the school curriculum in the UK, as well period products being distributed in schools. There is still so much that needs to change, but change *is* happening. Who knows what these unusual and increasingly popular types of activism will achieve next?

Fig. 45

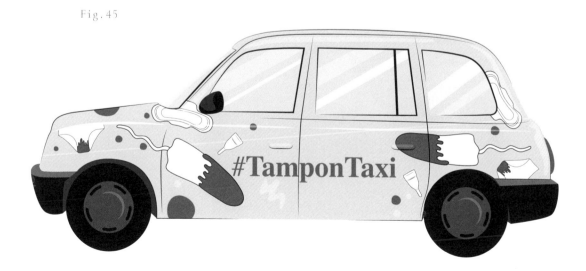

WHAT CAN I DO TO HELP?

The good news is that you — yes YOU, reading this book — can help make a change. Anyone can! One of the simplest things you can do today to help banish the shame surrounding menstruation is simply to talk about it more. Normalizing discussion about periods can only be good. It can help minimize dismissal of PMS symptoms that often lead to conditions going undiagnosed for years. It can also educate people, which in turn could help developing countries eradicate practices that put many in great danger. Creating a more open, compassionate and — most importantly — public conversation could do a lot to improve overall awareness of reproductive health. Breaking the cycle of keeping these things hidden and adopting inclusive language go hand-in-hand, and are basic first steps. Change is possible and we're slowly getting there, so don't ever stop talking about your period. I know I won't.

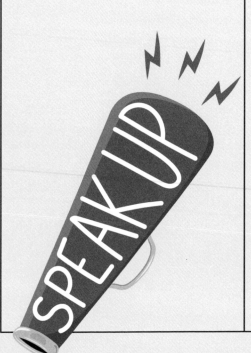

WAYS YOU CAN MAKE A DIFFERENCE

- Donate period products to local food banks and shelters.
- Seek out charities and find out how to support them, whether it's through donating, campaigning with them or spreading the good word (you'll find some listed on pages 182—85).
- Whether it's buying pads from an Amazon Wish List, sponsoring a run or helping a charity raise money, fundraisers and drives are always happening.
- If you can't provide support financially, do what you can to spread awareness. Never underestimate a simple retweet! It's a great way to signal boost and reach others who may have extra cash.
- Stock bathrooms with period products free of charge and, in the interest of inclusivity, stock *all* your bathrooms — be they men's, women's or gender neutral.
- Continue to educate yourself. Read up about what's happening in other countries, follow period-related news and talk to people about it.
- Buy products that are produced fairly. Support brands who donate a percentage of sales to charities or give products to those in need.
- The only influence most of us have is our voice and money, so try to make conscious choices when you shop if you can.
- Think about how you can you use your platform and speak out. Keep the topic on everyone's mind.

A
TOOL

PERIOD
KIT

Period Hacks

If you've reached the end of this book feeling ready to make a change, be it through taking action or simply altering the way you view menstruation, I'm so glad! Shifting your perspective and drawing new conclusions can be empowering, exhilarating and exhausting all at once, which is why I've put together a toolkit of sorts for you. From tips and tricks on how to manage your own period to a list of helpful resources, here are some of the things I definitely wish I had known sooner, lovingly passed from me to you.

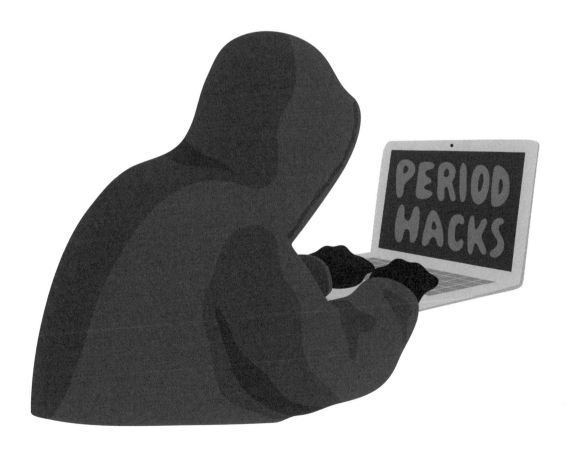

How to Track a Cycle

Fig. 46

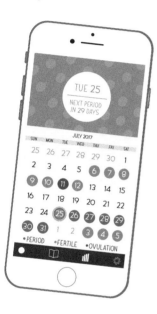

If there's one thing I hope this book has inspired you to do, it's track your cycle (Fig. 46). If not, here's one last list of benefits: it can help you understand certain patterns and find out when you're fertile, learn more about your over-all health, and understand and manage your mood. It's one thing to make this decision, but how do you actually start?

As we covered in the very first chapter, the beginning of a new cycle is the first day of your period (if you're somebody who experi-ences spotting, the first day of your cycle would be the first day you experience a flow of consistent bleeding), and the last day of your cycle is the day before your *next* period begins. So if you're mid–flow right now or have no idea what point you're at in your cycle, don't sweat it. Just wait until your next period.

The easiest way to keep track of your period, especially for the first time, is to simply write down when it starts and when it stops. Marking the days of the month you're bleeding should help you an-ticipate when you're likely to get your period the following month. This could be in a planner you carry around, in the notes section on your phone or even on the household calendar like we did at my family home (growing up, my mum would write 'TP' for 'Tara Period', then 'TP over' when it ended). Whenever something was wrong, or we were PMSing (it can be tough growing up in a household where multiple people are PMSing at once), she'd encourage us to check the calendar and count 28 days to see how far off our periods would be. The more we did this, the more we were able to grasp what our cycle lengths were. Little did we realize that my cycle would just do whatever the hell it wanted, but you get the idea. Mark the days your period is here; begin counting on the first day of bleeding (which is known as cycle day one) and go on to the first day of your next period, and voila — you have your cycle length.

Once you *really* get into it — and, trust me, you will — you can start tracking other things like PMS symptoms, changes in cervical fluid, sex drive status and all sorts! Tracking cervical fluid in particular is vital for those who want to monitor fertility (you can refer back to the list of changes and what they signify in the first chapter). If this sounds like an overwhelming task, fortunately, technology is in our favour. There are some wonderful apps out there you can use to track your cycle, and they definitely do way more than just track your period:

- Clue (available on iOS and Android)
- Eve (available on iOS and Android)
- Moody Month (available on iOS)
- Kindara (available on iOS and Android)
- Flo (available on iOS and Android)
- Ovia Fertility (available on iOS and Android)

I am particularly fond of Clue and Eve, as they have so many options for keeping track of PMS symptoms. Clue is a great educational resource, too, posting a number of insightful articles on their blog and social media feeds. The Eve app is almost like the BuzzFeed of periods — it comes with a whole community, quizzes and forums. I like how positive (although sometimes heavily gendered) their push notifications are: there's even one that reminds you to stock up on snacks! There is also other reproductive-health-focused tech out there on the market, such as basal body temperature (BBT) thermometers with corresponding apps. The idea is that the more information you input, the more accurate the predictions become. However, apps cannot predict what your body is going to do with 100 per cent accuracy. They're good for storing information in one place, and allow you to gain a better understanding of how a cycle works.

If tech isn't your thing and you want something simpler, here's how I track my periods in my journal (Fig. 47):

Fig. 47

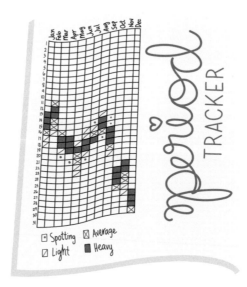

If you're doing this with pen and paper but struggle with maths, the brand Always has a period calculator on its website: always. co.uk/en-gb/period-calculator.

So, when does noting all this come in handy? Whenever your energy levels drop; when you feel particularly anxious out of nowhere; when you want to eat everything in sight; when you're incredibly horny; when your patience is wearing thin ... when *doesn't* it come in handy?! Although a period cannot be blamed for everything (sorry), the more you track how you feel as it approaches or during certain parts of your cycle, the less you'll be blindsided by your body's reactions. Over the years, I have made note of when I'm likely to be easily irritated and always try to schedule around that. This could mean moving a phone call or trying to reply to an irksome email when I'm feeling calmer. Of course, this isn't always possible, but it's good to keep in mind. Similarly, I try to avoid plans on day two of my period because I know I won't want to do anything; for me it's a day of rest. I also like to know when I'm going to feel extra sensitive physically, so I can avoid things like having my sore gums jabbed at the dentist or attempting to shape my eyebrows — although it's been years and I still haven't been able to sync my eyebrows with my uterus.

If your period is different each cycle or irregular, you should still write down notes. With so many people struggling to be taken seriously by healthcare providers, this is a great way to put your case forward. Remember, your period should not be leaving you in excruciating pain every month. While pain is common, it should not be so intense it makes you throw up or faint. Also, if over-the-counter pain relief medication does nothing, get it investigated. Track the days you feel pain and how you try to relieve it and whether it works before seeing someone. Try to implement a pain scale. Here's an example:

1   Manageable
2   A dull background ache
3   Distracting
4   So painful you have to pause
5   Unbearable, so you need to schedule
     around it / cancel plans

If you're somebody who experiences heavy bleeding, make a note of each day you're bleeding (especially if it's outside of your period), how often you're changing your products and how many products a day you're using. Do you soak a tampon or pad within the hour? Does your cup fill up quickly? Do your periods last longer than seven days? Do you experience spotting or bleeding in between periods? These are all things your healthcare provider will want to know. If you're not quite sure what qualifies as a heavy period or you want to check, the NHS has a 'Heavy Periods Self-Assessment' quiz available on their website (they've updated it to include menstrual cups). It calculates a heaviness rating on a scale of 1 to 18 and collates a list of bullet points that, if you live in the UK, can be printed and handed straight to a doctor: nhs.uk/conditions/heavy-periods/.

How to Manage Period Pain

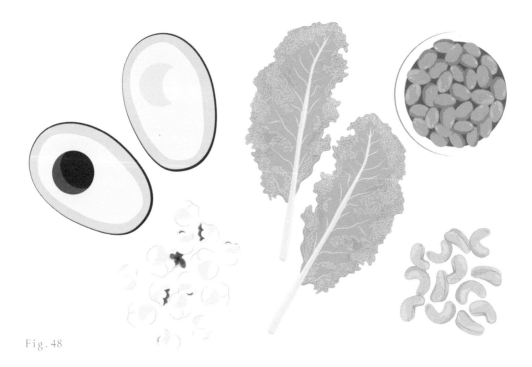

Fig. 48

When it comes to managing PMS symptoms, I have found the best way is to focus on diet and lifestyle changes. No, I don't mean dieting — you probably feel fed up enough as it is bleeding and cramping; you don't need the misery of a restrictive diet on top of that! But I do think it's worth being aware of what food and drink can help versus what can't. In recent years, the effectiveness of magnesium has been demonstrated in numerous studies and clinical trials, with evidence suggesting that magnesium deficiency may play an important role in several clinical conditions concerning reproductive health, such as premenstrual syndrome, dysmenorrhea and postmenopausal symptoms. Dr Lara Briden put this in simpler terms when writing for the app Clue: 'Magnesium calms the nervous system. The result is less anxiety, less cortisol and a better capacity to cope with stress. Reduced stress can, in turn, have positive effects on your menstrual cycle and health.' Great, sign me up!

Here are a list of foods that are rich in magnesium and worth eating more of in the run-up to your period (Fig. 48):

- Dark leafy greens like spinach and kale
- Avocado
- Sesame and pumpkin seeds
- Almond and cashew nuts
- Dark chocolate (70 per cent and above) or raw cacao
- Popcorn
- Tofu
- Baked beans
- Peanut butter

It's also been suggested that increasing your iron intake before and during a period can't hurt either, as you could potentially replace what you've lost. If you eat red meat, chances are you already get enough iron in your diet. For vegans and veggies alike, the list of iron-rich foods is similar to the above, with spinach, tofu and cashews being top of the chart again. Other good foods include beans and lentils, fortified breakfast cereals, oats and brown rice, as well as wholegrain and enriched breads.

You don't have to cut out carbs during this time. In fact, Dr Linda Bradley recommends eating 'complex' ones: 'Foods that have complex carbohydrates consist of three or more natural sugars and are rich in fibre. These foods enter the bloodstream gradually, causing only a moderate rise in insulin levels, which can help stabilize your mood.' She recommends foods such as sweet potatoes, squash, pumpkin, lentils and unprocessed oats.

Is there anything you need to avoid? While I don't want to tell you what you can or can't eat or drink during this time, it has been suggested that caffeine can increase discomfort from cramps and bloating. Dr Lori Shemek states, 'Caffeine is a vasoconstrictor; it makes blood vessels constrict and may cause the vessels that feed the uterus to tighten.' Feel like you can't function without carbonated drinks while you're bleeding? Me neither! Try switching to caffeine-free ones instead. Coffee fiend? Again, switch to something caffeine-free if you think this could be making cramps worse. Caffeine has also been linked to greater tenderness and making you more irritable. Chamomile tea is a good replacement because it has properties that may help relieve muscle spasms, which could reduce the severity of cramps. If herbal teas aren't your bag, you could always try decaf. Ultimately, eat and drink more of the stuff that brings you comfort during this time. I have to have a pizza every period, no exceptions allowed!

In terms of lifestyle changes, I'm not suggesting anything drastic. Using your period as a time to check in with yourself and tune in to what you really need is a good idea. Things like reducing stress and getting plenty of rest are great to try doing more of during this time, especially since there is a chance you're going to feel quite drained anyway. Of course, it won't always be possible, but don't feel bad. During most periods I'm a frantic, sleep-deprived, weepy mess. Just try adding in some time to do things that can help you relax, or try to avoid things that make you annoyed. For example, one of my favourite things to do is have a nice, long, hot bath and avoid social media for the night. Bonus tip: take an Epsom salts bath; they have magnesium sulphate in them. Heat in general is always a good idea, as it's very effective for relieving muscle tension and pain. Try using a heat pad or hot water bottle on your lower abdomen to relax the muscles; it doesn't matter if you have to keep reheating it. If you're feeling super emotional, why not embrace it and have a cathartic cry? We all have a bank of films that are guaranteed to make us lose it.

Here are some other ways you can try to relieve pain:

- Painkillers
- Changing into something comfortable
- Light exercise, like walking or yoga
- Have an orgasm
- Rest

There's no right or wrong way to get through a period. You've got to do whatever works for you!

How to Make Your Own Period Kit

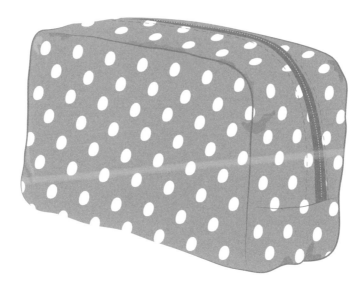

My mum was really great in terms of preparing me for my first peri-od. Not only was she able to warn me about it before it happened, she also made sure I had the products I needed. She handed me a bright, polka-dot makeup bag (which I still own to this day) full of items for me to try and get my head around. This period kit of sorts is something I've kept going all these years and definitely recom-mend. It makes menstruation just a little less stressful knowing all your products are in one place. Here are some things you could keep in yours:

- Period products of choice
- Pain relief
- Comfy underwear
- A smaller bag for when you're on the go (I really recommend a wet bag if you use wearable reusable products; many have two sections so you can keep the clean products separate from the used ones)

Other products I always try to have in the house are disposable heat pads and a stain remover, both of which are total lifesavers!

There's a lot of information out there about reusables, but not enough that focuses on how to obtain and start using them — so, please enjoy this mini guide.

MENSTRUAL CUPS

There are a multitude of extraordinary cups out there suited to different vaginas, menstrual flows and individual needs. This is why it can sometimes be hard to advise others on which cup they should try. Some cups sit low and some are designed with higher-sitting cervixes (represent!) in mind. Others are designed on a flow basis (heavy; average) and some are marketed by material (firm; soft). It's really about finding what works for you, and this search can sometimes take a substantial amount of time and money. However, there are a couple of things you can do to help you achieve that Goldilocks moment.

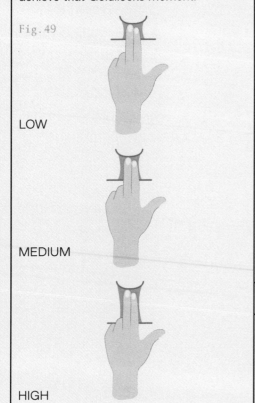

Fig. 49

LOW

MEDIUM

HIGH

First, try measuring your cervix (Fig. 49) to get a better understanding of its height. After you've washed your hands, find a comfortable position that will allow you to insert a finger with ease (I find squatting easiest). Once you're comfortable, slowly slide your middle or index finger into your vagina as far as you can. Try to relax your muscles while you do this. Use an in-and-upward motion and be careful not to scratch yourself. To 'measure' the height of your cervix, simply make note of how far your finger was inserted. For example, if you didn't have to reach much further than under your nail, you have a low cervix, as shown here. Don't expect to understand what you're feeling at first; it's something that requires practice and patience. As your cervix changes position subtly and frequently, try checking your cervical position every few days. Once you have a good idea of your height, you can narrow down what cups might work for you.

If you're not comfortable doing this, the team behind Put A Cup In It, a great source of information for menstrual cups, have a quiz you can take. It's pretty quick and designed to help you select the right cup for your body, age, activity level and so on, and it's available in different languages too: putacupinit.com/quiz.

A number of brands say it can take up to three cycles to determine whether or not their cup is right for you, so try not to feel too disheartened. There's a wide range out there if you don't get on with one brand and want to keep trying. Sometimes you just know when a product isn't for you and that's okay too.

CLOTH PADS

Before purchasing there are a few things you should consider, such as what your flow is like. Is it heavy? Is it light? Does it start off heavy and then become light? Think about what kind of absorbency you need. For example, it wouldn't make much sense owning a bunch of pads for a heavy flow when you have a light one, and vice versa. You'll also want to think about sizing; the best way to figure out what you need is to look at the disposable products that have worked for you in the past. You could measure them with a ruler and search for something similar. Most retailers will include information such as absorbency and size of the cloth pad (in either inches or centimetres) for each individual listing. It's likely they'll have a size chart on their website somewhere which you can consult to find a comparable item. Do this for different length pads if you wear a variety during your cycle.

If you've never worn disposable pads before and have no idea where to start with cloth pads, a lot of retailers carry starter kits. Consider them an introduction to cloth pads; they will normally include a variety of sizes. For example, Earthwise Girls stock a kit that contains seven pads: three mini, three regular, two heavy. They can range anywhere from duos to a kit of 12; it depends on how many you want. Some may even include wet bags you can keep them in. These come in handy when travelling or when you're unable to wash them immediately. This is a good place to begin, as it can help make the transition from disposables to cloth pads less overwhelming. You could also start your collection by buying a couple of pads in different brands and styles/shapes, allowing you to get a feel for what works without having to spend a lot of money when you're still unsure.

BUILDING COLLECTIONS AND WHAT TO DO IN THE MEANTIME

When it comes to reusable period products, it's likely the transition will take a few months. I have found this especially true of products like cloth pads and different forms of period underwear. With cloth pads in particular, approximately 15 to 25 are recommended (although you may need more depending on your flow and how often you change). In terms of pricing, it's not the same as going out and buying packs of disposables. You're often buying individual items (that last) at a higher price, so it can take a while to build a collection. If you have used disposables before, think about how many times you would change a day; that's the number you want to aim for.

CLEANING TIPS

One thing that can be slightly overwhelming about reusable period products is figuring out how to clean them. Here are some tips that have never let me down.

MENSTRUAL CUPS

I clean my menstrual cup after each use and after each cycle. Day-to-day, I simply empty it while I'm still sitting on the toilet and rinse it in the sink if there's residue. Sometimes I go straight to the sink if I want to keep an eye on roughly how much blood I'm losing. If you're unable to get to a sink between changes, toilet paper works fine too. You can just give it a good rinse when you get home. If you don't want to wait that long you could bring a bottle of water into the cubicle with you, but you don't have to.

In between cycles I sterilize my cup by boiling it in a pot on the stove (Fig. 50) for about 15 minutes. Again, different brands recommend different times, so always check. Every time my period ends I say I'm going to boil my cups so I'm better prepared for next time, but I always somehow forget to. It's a good tip, though, if you can get into the habit. But if you're unable to boil your cup, no worries — there are other ways you can clean it, such as using sterilizing solution or tablets. Some brands also sell their own cleaning products and devices. For example, Ruby Cup sell Ruby Clean, a foldable device you put in the microwave to clean your cup.

CLOTH PADS

1   Pre-treat cloth pads with fabric stain remover and leave for 10 minutes.
2   Once the treatment has soaked in/ isn't visible, fill a sink with cold water and leave the pads to soak for at least 20 minutes.
3   Wring them out and put them in the washing machine on a cold rapid wash using detergent, if you're doing them on their own. If you're adding them to a regular laundry cycle, put them in a wet bag so there's a bit of protection from fabric softener.
4   Leave to dry.

Avoid hot water, as it will encourage bloodstains to stay put, and try not to use fabric softeners, as they can make cloth pads less absorbent.

PERIOD UNDERWEAR

Different brands will recommend different cleaning methods, so always check their websites. If you're struggling to find instructions, here's a method I use which has worked on many brands:

1   Rinse your underwear as soon as you take it off; this will help get most of the blood out.
2   Pull the underwear inside out and run it under cold water.
3   Squeeze out excess water.
4   Put it on a cold wash, hold the fabric softener and use a delicates bag if you have one.
5   Hang dry, reuse and repeat!

Fig. 50

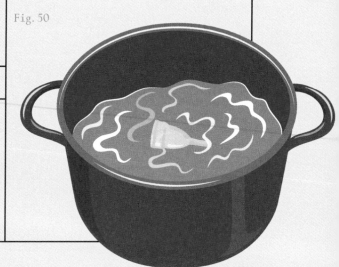

Inclusive Language

As we've touched upon, it's time for us to evolve beyond gender-specific language ('lady time'; 'feminine hygiene') when it comes to discussing menstruation. Using gender-neutral language is a basic courtesy that makes everyone feel included. There doesn't need to be a special word like 'menstruator' either, as you can just say 'people with periods' or 'those who menstruate' — y'know, terms I have been using throughout this entire book. You didn't even notice, did you? Gotcha!

Here are some really easy changes you can include in your language moving forward:

INSTEAD OF   REPLACE WITH

Sanitary products ⟶ Menstrual products
Feminine hygiene products ⟶ Period products
Becoming a woman ⟶ Starting puberty
Women's health ⟶ Reproductive health
Women and girls ⟶ People who menstruate
People who have periods
She/her ⟶ They/them

Resources

SUPPORT

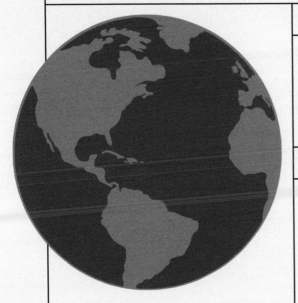

ADENOMYOSIS AND ENDOMETRIOSIS

AFRICA

GHANA
- Endometriosis Foundation Ghana
  endometriosisghana.org
- Endo Charity
  endometriosischarityghana.com

NIGERIA
- Endometriosis Support Group
  esgn.org

SOUTH AFRICA
- Foundation for Endometriosis
  Awareness, Advocacy and Support
  facebook.com/endoawarenessct

ASIA

INDIA
- Endometriosis Society of India
  endosocind.org

JAPAN
- Japan Endometriosis Association
  jemanet.org

AUSTRALIA
- The Endometriosis Association
  qendo.org.au
- EndoActive Australia & NZ
  endoactive.org.au
- Endometriosis Australia
  endometriosisaustralia.org

CENTRAL AMERICA

BARBADOS
- Barbados Association of
  Endometriosis & PCOS
  endoandpcosbb.com

MEXICO
- Endometriosis Mexico
  endometriosismexico.com

TRINIDAD AND TOBAGO
- Trinidad & Tobago
  Endometriosis Association
  endott.org

EUROPE

AUSTRIA
- Endometriose Vereinigung Austria
  eva-info.at

BELGIUM
- EndoHome – Endometriosis
  Association Belgium
  endohome.be

DENMARK
- Endometriose Foreningen Denmark
  endo.dk

FINLAND
- Korento ry
  korento.fi

FRANCE
- EndoFrance
  endofrance.org

- ENDOmind France
  endomind.org
- Mon Endométriose
  Ma Souffrance Métropole
  mon-endo-ma-souffrance.fr

GERMANY
- Endometriose-Vereinigung
  Deutschland e.V.
  endometriose-vereinigung.de

HUNGARY
- "Együtt könnyebb" Női
  Egészségért Alapítvány
  noiegeszsegert.hu

ICELAND
- Samtök um Endómetríósu
  endo.is

ITALY
- Associazione Italiana Endometriosi
  endoassoc.it
- Associazione Progetto Endometriosi
  apeonlus.com

NETHERLANDS
- Endometriose Stichting
  endometriose.nl

NORWAY
- Endometriose Foreningen Norge
  endometriose.no

POLAND
- Pierwszy Polski Portal
  o Endometriozie
  endometrioza.org
- Polksie Stowarzyszenie Endometrioza
  pse.aid.pl

PORTUGAL
- MulherEndo — Associação
  Portuguesa de Apoio a Mulheres
  com Endometriose
  mulherendo.pt

ROMANIA
- Asociația Eu și Endometrioza
  eusiendometrioza.ro
- Asociatia SOS Endometrioza
  facebook.com/EndoLady

SPAIN
- Asociación de Endometriosis
  de Madrid
  endomadrid.org
- Asociacion de
  Endometriosis España
  endoinfo.org
- Endometriosis Catalunya
  endometriosiscatalunya.com

SWEDEN
- Endometriosföreningen Sverige
  endometriosforeningen.com

SWITZERLAND
- Endo-Help
  endo-help.ch

TURKEY
- Turkish Society for Endometriosis
  and Adenomyosis
  endometriozisdernegi.org
- Turkish Society for Pelvic Pain
  and Endometriosis
  paed.org.tr

NORTH AMERICA

CANADA
- The Endometriosis Network Canada
  endometriosisnetwork.ca

PUERTO RICO
- Fundación Puertorriqueña
  de Pacientes con Endometriosis
  endometriosispr.net

UNITED STATES
- Endometriosis Association
  endometriosisassn.org
- Endometriosis Foundation of America
  endofound.org

- Endometriosis Research Center
  endocenter.org

UK & IRELAND

- Endometriosis Association of Ireland
  endo.ie
- Endometriosis UK
  endometriosis-uk.org

FIBROIDS

EUROPE

FRANCE
- Fibrome Info France
  fibrome-info-france.org

NORTH AMERICA

- The Fibroid Foundation
  fibroidfoundation.org
- Fibroid Relief
  fibroidrelief.org
- National Uterine Fibroids Foundation
  nuff.org

UK AND IRELAND

- British Fibroid Trust
  britishfibroidtrust.org.uk
- Fibroid Network
  fibroid.network

POLYCYSTIC OVARY SYNDROME

INDIA

- Conquer PCOS
  conquerpcos.org

NORTH AMERICA

- Insulite Health PCOS
  pcos.com
- The National Polycystic Ovary
  Syndrome Association
  pcoschallenge.com

- PCOS Awareness Association
  pcosaa.org

UK & IRELAND

- Verity
  verity-pcos.org.uk

PREMENSTRUAL DYSPHORIC DISORDER

NORTH AMERICA

- International Association
  for Premenstrual Disorders
  iapmd.org

UK & IRELAND

- Mind
  mind.org.uk/information-support/
  types-of-mental-health-problems/
  premenstrual-dysphoric-
  disorder-pmdd/#.XcqaEZL7TOQ
- National Association for
  Premenstrual Syndrome
  pms.org.uk
- Vicious Cycle: Making PMDD Visible
  viciouscyclepmdd.com

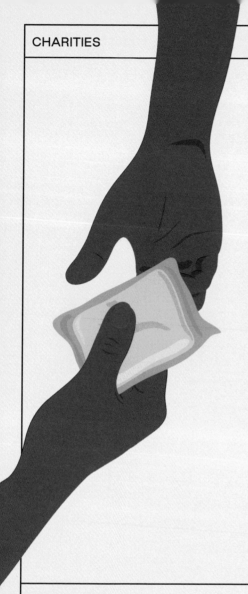

AFRICA

- The African Coalition for Menstrual Health Management
  twitter.com / AfriCoMHM

  ### ETHIOPIA
- Dignity Period
  dignityperiod.org
- Ethiopiaid Ireland
  ethiopiaid.ie

  ### KENYA
- Huru
  huruinternational.org

  ### MALAWI
- Supreme Sanitary Pads
  suprememalawi.com

  ### NIGERIA
- Health Aid for All Initiative
  hafai.org

  ### RWANDA
- SHE Enterprises
  sheinnovates.com

  ### SIERRA LEONE
- One Girl
  onegirl.org.au

  ### SOUTH AFRICA
- Girl Movement
  girlmovement.co.za

  ### UGANDA
- AFRIpads
  afripadsfoundation.org
- Girl Power Pads
  twitter.com / GirlPowerUg
- WoMena
  womena.dk

  ### ZIMBABWE
- Sanitary Aid Zimbabwe
  twitter.com / SanitaryZ

INTERNATIONAL

- Binti International
  bintiperiod.org / take-action
- Empowering Women Period.
  empoweringwomenperiod.org
- HappyPeriod
  hashtaghappyperiod.org
- Hygiene and You
  hygieneandyou.com
- Mino Period
  minoperiod.com
- Your Time Foundation
  yourtimefoundation.com

AUSTRALIA	• KidsCan kidscan.org.nz/our-work/ health-for-kids
• The Clams (donations at events) theclams.com.au (Melbourne) • Ethiopiaid Australia ethiopiaid.org.au • The Period Project theperiodproject.org.au • The Rough Period theroughperiod.org (New South Wales) • Share the Dignity sharethedignity.com.au/axethetax	• kidspot kidspot.co.nz/health/ tacking-action-period-poverty • Shine 2shine.org.nz/i-want-to-help- others/donating-items (Auckland) • SPINZS spinzs.co.nz • United Sustainable Sisters tamakiwrap.org.nz/projects-1

CANADA	**UK & IRELAND**
• Ethiopiaid Canada ethiopiaid.ca • Femme International femmeinternational.org • Mother Nature Partnership mothernaturepartnership.org • Pads4Girls lunapads.com/pages/pads4girls • The Period Purse theperiodpurse.com • Red Bindi Organization for Menstrual Health redbindi.org	• Irise International irise.org.uk • Plan International UK plan-uk.org • The Red Box Project redboxproject.org ENGLAND Bolton • Fresh as a Daisy BL twitter.com/bolton_daisy Brighton • The Homeless Period Brighton facebook.com/ thehomelessperiodbrighton
INDIA	Cornwall • Street Cramps streetcramps.org Croydon • We-Stap we-stap.com Lancashire • FemCura facebook.com/FemcuraUK • Free Period UK twitter.com/freeperioduk London • Bloody Good Period bloodygoodperiod.com • Period. twitter.com/PeriodCharity
• Aakar Innovations aakarinnovations.com • The Pad Project thepadproject.org • Pasand pasand.org • SheWings shewings.com • Shomota shomota.com	
NEW ZEALAND	
• Dignity dignitynz.com • Feel Good Period facebook.com/fgperiod (Wellington)	

Manchester
- The Crimson Wave
  twitter.com/CrimsonWaveOrg
- Every Month
  everymonthcampaign.org
- Poverty in Periods
  povertyinperiods.wordpress.com

Milton Keynes
- Girl Pack MK
  twitter.com/GirlPackMK

Sevenoaks
- The Hygiene Bank
  twitter.com/thehygienebank

Sheffield
- The Homeless Period
  Appeal Sheffield
  facebook.com/homelessperiodappeal

Southampton
- The Homeless Period
  thehomelessperiodsouthampton.
  weebly.com

South Tyneside
- The Period Poverty Project
  facebook.com/
  theperiodpovertyproject

Staffordshire
- Period Power
  twitter.com/PeriodPower2

Stevenage
- A Bloody Good Cause
  abloodygoodcause.wordpress.com

Wolverhampton
- The Homeless Period Wolverhampton
  facebook.com/
  homelessperiodwolverhampton

Wrexham
- WINGS Wrexham
  facebook.com/wingswrexham

York
- The Lunar Project
  facebook.com/lunarprojectyork

IRELAND
- Stop Period Poverty Ireland
  facebook.com/
  groups/1901513276810770

NORTHERN IRELAND
- Another World Belfast
  anotherworldbelfast.com
- The Homeless Period Belfast
  facebook.com/
  TheHomelessPeriodBelfast
- The Homeless Period Mid Ulster
  facebook.com/
  homelessperiodmidulster

SCOTLAND
- Hey Girls UK
  heygirls.co.uk

Edinburgh
- Bleedin' Saor
  bleedinsaor.com
- The Homeless Period Edinburgh
  facebook.com/
  homelessperiodedinburgh
- Simon Community Period
  Friendly Points
  simonscotland.org/period-friendly

WALES
- Periods in Poverty
  twitter.com/DignityCaerdydd

USA

- Days for Girls
  daysforgirls.org
- Girls Helping Girls Period
  girlshelpinggirlsperiod.org

Georgia (Atlanta)
- Code Red
  coderedco.org

Massachusetts (Boston)
- Hope and Comfort
  hopeandcomfort.org

Michigan (Lansing)
- Helping Women Period
  helpingwomenperiod.org

New Mexico (Albuquerque)
- Women2Be
  women2be.org

New York
- Project Pixie
  iheartprojectpixie.org (tri-state area)

- RACKET
  weracket.com (New York City)

Ohio (Cleveland)
- Period Partner
  periodpartner.org

Oregon (Portland)
- Periodic, Inc.
  periodicinc.com

Rhode Island (Providence)
- UnTabooed
  twitter.com/UnTabooed

South Carolina
- Homeless Period Project
  homelessperiodproject.org

Washington, DC
- BRAWS
  BRAWS.org
- I Support the Girls
  isupportthegirls.org

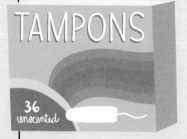

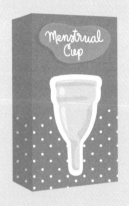

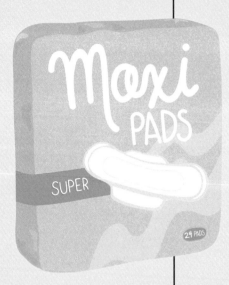

DISPOSABLE PADS AND TAMPONS

- **&SISTERS**
  andsisters.co.uk
- **Always**
  always.com
- **Bodyform**
  bodyform.co.uk
- **BON**
  bonlifestyle.com
- **Cora**
  cora.life
- **DAME**
  wearedame.co
- **DAYE**
  yourdaye.com
- **Flo**
  hereweflo.co
- **Freda**
  myfreda.com
- **Grace & Green**
  graceandgreen.co
- **Kind**
  kindorganic.com
- **Kotex**
  ubykotex.com
- **L Organic**
  thisisl.com

- **Lil-Lets**
  lil-lets.com
- **Lola**
  mylola.com
- **Natracare**
  natracare.com
- **o.b.**
  ob-tampons.com
- **OHNE**
  ohne.co
- **Oi**
  oi4me.com
- **Organyc**
  organyc-online.com
- **Playtex**
  playtexplayon.com
- **Rael**
  getrael.com
- **Seventh Generation**
  seventhgeneration.com
- **Tampax**
  tampax.com
- **TOTM**
  totm.com
- **Veeda**
  veeda.co.uk
- **Yoni**
  yoni.care

REUSABLE PADS

- Babipur
  babipur.co.uk/reusable-menstrual-cups-pads.html
- Bloom & Nora
  bloomandnora.com
- Boobalou
  boobalou.co.uk
- Cheeky Mama
  cheekywipes.com
- Crimson Moon
  crimsonmooncsp.com
- Domino Pads
  dominopads.com
- Earthwise Girls
  earthwisegirlsuk.co.uk
- Eco Dreams
  ecodreams.co.uk
- Eco Femme
  ecofemme.org
- Eco Rainbow
  ecorainbow.co.uk
- Honour Your Flow
  honouryourflow.co.uk
- ImseVimse
  imsevimse.co.uk
- LaliPads
  lalicup.com
- Lunapads
  lunapads.com
- Moon Times
  moontimes.co.uk
- Precious Stars
  preciousstars.co.uk
- TCS Eco
  tcs-eco.co.uk

MENSTRUAL CUPS AND DISCS; SOFTCUPS

- AmyCup
  amycup.com
- Blossom
  blossomcup.com
- Cora Cup
  cora.life
- Cotton Mermaid
  cottonmermaid.com
- DivaCup
  divacup.com
- Dot
  dotforall.com
- Femmecup
  femmecup.com
- FemmyCycle
  femmycycle.com
- Fleurcup
  fleurcup.com
- FLEX
  flexfits.com
- Fun Cup
  thefuncup.com
- Genial Day
  genialday.com
- Hello
  thehellocup.com
- Hey Girls
  heygirls.co.uk
- JuJu Cup
  juju.com.au
- Keeper
  keeper.com
- LadyCup
  ladycup.eu
- LaliCup
  lalicup.com
- LENA
  lenacup.com
- LouLou
  en.louloucup.com
- Lunette
  lunette.com
- Luv Ur Body
  luvur-body.com
- Lybera
  lybera.com
- Merula
  merula-cup.de/en
- Mooncup
  mooncup.co.uk
- OrganiCup
  organicup.com
- Saalt
  saaltco.com
- Sckoon Cup
  sckoon.com

- Selena
  selenacup.com
- Shecup
  shecup.com
- Si-Bell
  sibellmenstrualcup.com
- Silja
  silja-cup.com
- Super Jennie
  superjennie.com
- Sustain Natural
  sustainnatural.com
- Tampax Cup
  tampaxcup.com
- Tieutcup
  tieut.com
- Tulip Cup
  thetulipcup.com
- UltuCup
  ultucup.com

PERIOD UNDERWEAR

- Dear Kate
  dearkate.com
- Flux
  fluxundies.com
- LaliPanties
  lalicup.com
- Luna Undies
  lunapads.com
- Modibodi
  modibodi.co.uk
- Ruby Love
  rubylove.com
- THINX
  shethinx.com
- WUKA
  wuka.co.uk

SUBSCRIPTION SERVICES

- Aunt Flow
  goauntflow.com
- Blume
  blume.com
- Bonjour Jolie
  bonjourjolie.com
- Cora
  cora.life
- Daye
  yourdaye.com
- Freda
  myfreda.com
- Flux
  fluxundies.com
- Kali
  kaliboxes.com
- L Organic
  thisisl.com
- Lola
  mylola.com
- Monthlies
  monthlies.co.uk
- OHNE
  ohne.co
- Pink Parcel
  pink-parcel.com
- Sustain Natural
  sustainnatural.com
- TOTM
  totm.com

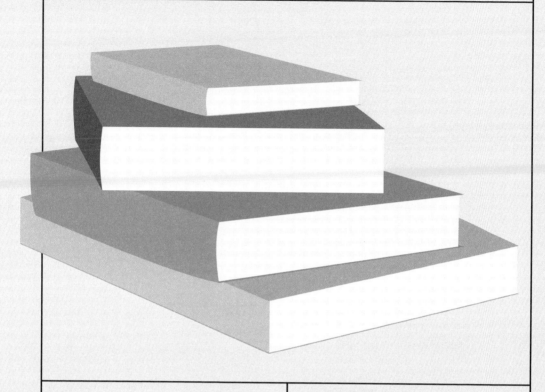

BOOKS

- Baker, Claire
  50 Things You Need to Know About Periods: Know Your Flow and Live in Sync with Your Cycle (Pavilion Books, 2020).
- Barnett, Emma
  Period. (HQ, 2019).
- Byrne, Natalie
  Period. (Break the Habit Press, 2018).
- Dahlqvist, Anna
  It's Only Blood: Shattering the Taboo of Menstruation (Zed Books, 2018).
- Enright, Lynn
  Vagina: A Re-Education (Allen & Unwin, 2019).
- Gunter, Dr Jen
  The Vagina Bible: The Vulva and the Vagina — Separating the Myth from the Medicine (Piatkus, 2019).
- Hill, Maisie
  Period Power: Harness Your Hormones and Get Your Cycle Working For You (Green Tree, 2019).
- Okamoto, Nadya
  Period Power: A Manifesto for the Menstrual Movement (Simon & Schuster Books for Young Readers, 2018).
- Steward, Robyn
  The Autism-Friendly Guide to Periods (Jessica Kingsley Publishers, 2019).
- Weiss-Wolf, Jennifer
  Periods Gone Public: Taking a Stand for Menstrual Equity (Arcade Publishing, 2017).
- Witton, Hannah
  The Hormone Diaries: The Bloody Truth About Our Periods (Wren & Rook, 2019).

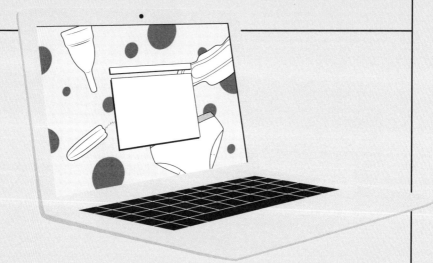

CAMPAIGNS

- #FreePeriods
  freeperiods.org
- Betty for Schools
  bettyforschools.co.uk
- The Cup Effect
  thecupeffect.org
- Free the Tampons
  freethetampons.org
- The Homeless Period
  thehomelessperiod.com
- PERIOD. The Menstrual Movement
  period.org
- Period Positive
  periodpositive.com
- The Period Poverty Project
  theperiodpovertyproject.com
- Project Period
  thisisourperiod.org
- Red Dot
  reddotcampaign.org

HEAVY PERIODS & CONDITIONS

- National Institute for Health
  and Care Excellence
  nice.org.uk
- Wear White Again
  wearwhiteagain.co.uk

REPRODUCTIVE HEALTH

- Clue
  helloclue.com
- Let's Talk Period
  letstalkperiod.ca
- Society for Menstrual
  Cycle Research
  menstruationresearch.org
- Wellbeing of Women
  wellbeingofwomen.org.uk
- Women's Health Concern
  womens–health–concern.org

REUSABLE PRODUCTS

- The Green Vagina
  thegreenvagina.com
- Menstrual Cup Reviews
  menstrualcupreviews.net
- The Period Blog
  theperiodblog.com
- Put a Cup In It
  putacupinit.com
- Reusable Menstrual Products
  clothpads.wordpress.com

Biographies

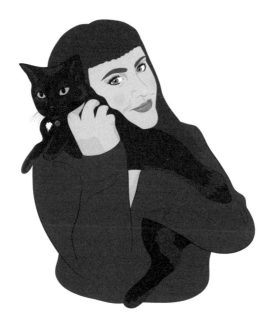

Tara Costello is a social media manager and writer who is passionate about challenging stigma and making taboo topics more inclusive. Residing in London with her fierce familiar, Buffy, she's never been afraid to stand up and speak about things she thinks are important. In 2015, she was one of the people who led the viral response to the controversial Protein World advertising campaign in tube stations, which received a lot of media coverage and was the subject of various university lectures, as well as leading to a spot on *Stylist's* 'Fearless Feminists of 2015' list. It also prompted the London mayor to ban all body-shaming media from the London Underground. She has since gone on to found and manage a number of award-winning (and -losing) blogs; in 2015, she was shortlisted for 'Best Relationship & Sex Blog' at *Cosmopolitan's* Blog Awards and shortlisted again the following year for 'Best Sex & Relationships Influencer'. In 2016, at the UK Blog Awards, a blog she co-founded was highly commended within the 'Education' category.

Although the blogs have come and gone, Tara has continued to write and tackle more difficult topics. She has been published by *The Huffington Post*, *Metro*, *Playboy*, *HelloGiggles* and more. Through her work, she hopes to inspire people from all walks of life to view periods differently.

Her favourite thing to do while menstruating is to watch a film in bed, surrounded by snacks, and have a good cry.

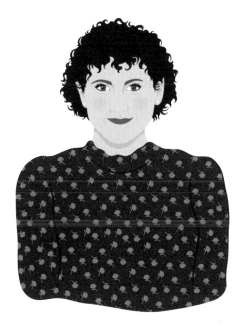

Mary Purdie is a digital illustrator based in Los Angeles, California. She pours her heart into her artwork with the goal of spreading positive and uplifting messages that encourage self–love, self–care and introspection. She is passionate about reproductive rights, and her illustrated poster on this topic was selected for a 2017 national–al touring art exhibition, Hear Our Voice. Mary's illustrations about miscarriage were published to accompany a story by the World Health Organization. She was also part of a creative campaign by the American Foundation for Suicide Prevention, and her piece was published in the *Washington Post*. She illustrated a book of poetry in 2019, written by Katie Zeppieri and titled *She Rises*, which aims to be a source of comfort for young women who struggle with anxiety.

Before and during menstruation, Mary craves spicy food and sweet desserts. She loves to snuggle with a cozy blanket and watch emotional movies that are sure to make her cry.

Acknowledgements

Tara Costello: There are a ton of people I'd like to thank for not only shaping me into the human I am today, but also helping me be able to pull this book off. In no particular order:

A special thanks to everyone I spoke to who shared their story with me, as well as those who contributed. You are the inspiration behind this book and why I wanted to write it.

I'd like to thank both my agent, Megan Carroll, and editor, Ali Gitlow, for all your dedication and diligence. Without you, this book would not have been possible. And of course, Mary Purdie, the wonderful person who illustrated this book. Thanks also to Nina Jua Klein for designing the book, and Martha Jay for copy-editing and proofreading it.

To my parents, for raising my sister and me in a household where no topics were off-limits and always encouraging us to ask questions and explore whatever we wanted to. Mum, thanks for entertaining my questions about the human body and giving me the sex talk several years earlier than you planned to. And most importantly, for preparing me for my period. Dad, thanks for allowing us to talk about such topics so openly and for never dismissing us, for the endless supply of period puns, and snack runs too. Sis, thanks for sharing the woes of PMS with me and the infamous lucky sani. And to the large amount of incredibly strong and resilient women in my bloodline.

To my ridiculously patient and supportive partner Iain, who has listened to many PMS-induced rants and always encouraged me to pursue my dreams, as well as boiling my cup or popping a wheat bag in the microwave, no questions asked.

To my amazing friends who have stuck by me while I'm growing through stuff, continuing to raise me up and shine with me. And to those who supported me throughout this project through many strops and meltdowns: Maisie, Sonia, Nadia, Steph, Cia, Aisling, Liv and probably a few more I'm forgetting. Sorry, I love you!

To the mega fluffs and the puff, Ozzie, Felix and Buffy. This cute trio of animals have supported me through many bad periods and days in bed.

And lastly to Rachel Bloom, who will probably never read this, for blessing us with the glorious 'Period Sex' song and validating all us menstruating hornbags.

Mary Purdie: Thank you to Tara Costello for writing this important book and allowing me to be a part of it! Thank you to Ali Gitlow for being so lovely to work with during this process and to Nina Jua Klein for her amazing design skills. Thanks also to our copy-editor Martha Jay.

Special thanks to my mom and sister for preparing me for my first period, and for approaching me after seeing my first maxi pad wrapper in the garbage — even though it was a false alarm. Thank you to my sister, Gretchen, for teaching me how to use a tampon for the first time by coaching me from the other side of the bathroom door, and for buying me my first menstrual cup. Thank you to both my parents and my sister for putting up with my PMS meltdowns from a young age and giving me space for those emotions to come out.

Thank you to my adoring husband, DeAndre, for always being willing to take me out for ice cream when the craving calls, and for loving me through my emotional rollercoaster rides.

Finally, thank you to every friend and stranger who has ever lent me a pad or tampon during an unexpected emergency in a public bathroom.

In respect to links in the book, Verlagsgruppe Random
House expressly notes that no illegal content was
discernible on the linked sites at the time the links were
created. The Publisher has no influence at all over the
current and future design, content or authorship of the
linked sites. For this reason Verlagsgruppe Random House
expressly disassociates itself from all content on linked
sites that has been altered since the link was created and
assumes no liability for such content.

Library of Congress Control Number: 2019947061

A CIP catalogue record for this book is available from
the British Library.

Editorial direction: Ali Gitlow
Copyediting: Martha Jay
Design and layout: Nina Jua Klein Studio
Production management: Friederike Schirge
Separations: Reproline Mediateam
Printing and binding: DZS Grafik, d.o.o., Ljubljana
Paper: Tauro Offset

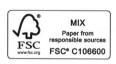

MIX
Paper from
responsible sources
FSC® C106600
FSC
www.fsc.org

Verlagsgruppe Random House FSC® N001967

Printed in Slovenia

ISBN 978-3-7913-8646-1

www.prestel.com